The Fast Food Diet

WITHDRAWN

The
Fast
Food
Diet

Lose Weight and Feel Great Even If You're Too Busy to Eat Right

STEPHEN SINATRA, M.D.,
and
JIM PUNKRE

Foreword by Barry Sears, Ph.D.

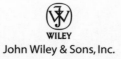

WILEY

John Wiley & Sons, Inc.

Published by John Wiley & Sons, Inc., Hoboken, New Jersey
Published simultaneously in Canada

Design and composiiton by Navta Associates, Inc.

The information contained in this book is not intended to serve as a replacement for pro-fessional medical advice. Any use of the information in this book is at the reader's discre-tion. The author and the publisher specifically disclaim any and all liability arising directly or indirectly from the use or application of any information contained in this book. A health care professional should be consulted regarding your specific situation.

For general information about our other products and services, please contact our Customer Care Department within the United States at (800) 762-2974, outside the United States at (317) 572-3993 or fax (317) 572-4002.

Wiley also publishes its books in a variety of electronic formats. Some content that appears in print may not be available in electronic books. For more information about Wiley products, visit our web site at www.wiley.com.

Library of Congress Cataloging-in-Publication Data:

Sinatra, Stephen T., date.
    The fast food diet : lose weight and feel great even if you're too busy to eat right / Stephen Sinatra and James Punkre ; foreword by Barry Sears.
        p. cm.
    Includes bibliographical references and index.
    ISBN 0-471-79047-8 (pbk.)
    1. Reducing diets—United States. 2. Weight loss—United States. 3. Convenience foods—Health aspects—United States. 4. Fast food restaurants—Health aspects—United States. 5. Food habits—United States.   I. Punkre, Jim. II. Title.
    RM222.2S555 2006
    613.2'5—dc22

                                                                    2006002082

Printed in the United States of America

10 9 8 7 6 5 4 3 2 1

This book is dedicated to the parents of America—and to their children, who are the hope of our country's healthy future.

We can end the obesity epidemic that is ruining America. Children learn by imitating their parents' actions. No matter what your socioeconomic-cultural level may be, your children will follow what you *do*, not merely what you say. If you set the example of choosing healthier foods and better nutrition in general, so will your children. You'll be giving them a gift that will last their entire lifetime, so they can enjoy a healthy life that is free of disease, suffering, prescription drugs, and premature death.

Stephen Sinatra, M.D.
Jim Punkre

CONTENTS

ACKNOWLEDGMENTS

To Jim Punkre, who gave me the idea for this book as well as his insightful ideas and tireless energy that helped make the book a reality.

To Matthew Hoffman for his research into the fast-food industry, Martina Punkre for her detailed editing, Debbie Del-Signore for keeping all the details straight, and Jeff Cox for his eagle eye.

To Tom Miller, our editor at John Wiley & Sons, for giving us the opportunity to help improve the way America eats.

To Bob Tuttle, who gave me the chance to manage his fast-food restaurant in Bellmore, New York, back in my high school years.

To my editorial, research, and marketing team for my monthly newsletter *Heart, Health & Nutrition* published by Healthy Directions in Potomac, Maryland.

To JoAnne Piazza, my trusted assistant and advisor.

To my sibs who grew up with me in Long Island: Pam, Dick, and Maria; and to their wonderful second families.

To all our children and grandchildren: Donna, Dan, Kristin, Brad, Greg, Jen, March, Step, Drew, Emma, Claire, Cecelia, and Cal.

To Jan Sinatra, my wife, best friend, late-night editor, lover, and life companion.

—Stephen Sinatra, M.D.
Jim Punkre

FOREWORD

The fast-food industry today is facing a tremendous challenge as well as an unprecedented opportunity. Fast food has been instrumental in conquering the problem of hunger in America. A warm meal is now so affordable and abundantly available that no one in our country should ever have to go hungry. The challenge the fast-food industry now faces is to make their meals more nutritious and calorie-conscious to benefit the health and weight of their customers.

We are eating more fast food in North America than ever before, and experts say this trend will not only continue but increase. Time and money constraints will force this upon us. Soon the lovingly prepared home-cooked meal of yesteryear will become the rare luxury that today's four-star restaurant experience now is. Faced with rising levels of obesity and diet-related health problems, the fast-food industry must accept the responsibility of providing more healthful and less fattening items on their menus. Their customers deserve a real choice. It is no coincidence that people who rely upon fast food for a significant portion of their diet are among the 40 percent of Americans who have inadequate or no health insurance. This unfortunate situation is unlikely to change any time soon, so Dr.

Sinatra's solution presented in this book is especially timely—and practical.

Dr. Steve Sinatra is one of the top preventive cardiologists in America. No one has a better understanding of the importance of food in preventing and reversing cardiovascular disorders and other degenerative diseases. The uniqueness of *The Fast Food Diet* is that Dr. Sinatra, instead of condemning the fast-food industry or pressuring it to change, is initiating this important transformation at the grassroots level. In *The Fast Food Diet*, he shows readers how to eat smarter and more nutritiously at any fast-food establishment so they will actually become healthier as they lose weight. What a brilliant strategy and practical approach!

This book is greatly needed because, while our daily life is ruled by time compression, our genes still herald from the Stone Age and rule our dietary desires. We are genetically conditioned to require small meals every four to six hours; a seemingly impossible task given today's lifestyle. Furthermore, our genes dictate a balance of protein, carbohydrate, and fat to provide the best hormonal response for weight control and overall wellness.

This is where fast food comes in. With a little know-how, you can always find protein in any fast-food restaurant. To maintain a healthy weight, you simply need to reduce the carbohydrates and sugars that accompany it to keep your appetite and insulin under control until your next meal. That's what this book will teach you. Once you master the simple tricks developed by Dr. Sinatra, you can indeed make use of fast food as a realistic alternative in times when you can't make the ideal choice.

There is much truth in the saying "You are what you eat." Steve Sinatra demonstrates that fast food can actually help you achieve your ultimate goal of continuing wellness.

—Barry Sears, Ph.D., author of *The Zone*

Get Smarter, Get Slimmer on Fast Food

America is a fast-food nation, for better and for worse. Consider the typical weekday. The alarm goes off and the family's bare feet start hitting the floor immediately. Everyone's probably running a little late because they didn't get enough sleep. (Americans sleep an average of seven hours a night, down from nine hours a century ago.) Getting the kids ready for school requires a Herculean effort: brushing teeth, washing faces, and digging under the couch for overdue library books. Time for a quick bowl of cereal? Probably not. So you rush out the door with an empty stomach. Maybe you'll snatch something on the way—or just do without anything to eat until lunch.

This frenetic pace doesn't let up at work. There's hardly such a thing as a lunch "hour" anymore. More likely you'll grab food at a take-out joint near the office and wolf it down on the way to the bank or some other errand. Then it's back to work until quitting time maybe five, six, or seven hours later. At that point your blood sugar is crashing and the last thing on your mind is cooking something from scratch. Ravenous and stressed-out from your day, you point the car to KFC or Wendy's or Burger King. You want something fast because you're practically starving and there's still the kids' homework to oversee, chores to do, and perhaps a game or your favorite TV show to catch before crashing into bed.

Fast food is so affordable and plentiful that millions of North Americans eat it every single day—or many times a week. We now eat on average five meals a week outside the home, in addition to snacking on convenience foods. The average adult consumes three hamburgers and four orders of fries every week. On any given day, 25 percent of all people in North America eat a fast-food meal. It's just so easy to hop in the car, zip the whole family through the drive-thru, and have dinner over and done in ten or fifteen minutes. No cooking, no cleanup, no stress—with time left over for errands and maybe some TV, plus change from a twenty-dollar bill.

But there is another side to fast food, a darker side that many people are now becoming aware of "the hard way," as we doctors say. We can no longer deny that all this fast food is making us fat. It is also making us sick. I've been called to the emergency room in the middle of the night to try to save a mom or dad who has just suffered a heart attack. I know kids who are nine, ten, eleven years of age who must inject themselves with insulin shots every day because they already have adult-onset, or Type 2 diabetes—something unheard of twenty years ago. Everywhere I look I see entire families in tragically overstuffed bodies, huffing and puffing just to carry their extra weight from the car to the sofa, to work and to school.

Nearly two-thirds of America's adults are currently overweight. One-third of the adult population is obese (officially defined as being 30 pounds overweight or more). Childhood obesity has reached alarming and epidemic proportions. Our passion for high-fat, high-salt, and high-calorie fast foods has become a major threat to our health. Consider these depressing facts:

- Type 2 diabetes is three times as common today as it was forty years ago, mainly because of our increasing weight. The link between obesity and diabetes is so strong that researchers have coined a new word, "diabesity," to describe it.

- Heart disease remains the leading killer of North Americans, largely due to elevated insulin and artery inflammation, both of which are caused by diets high in sugar and refined carbohydrates, as well as saturated and trans fats— the hallmarks of most fast foods.

- Deaths from breast cancer and prostate cancer in the United States dwarf the rates in countries where fast food isn't popular. Studies show that high-fat foods fuel the growth of many tumors, acting as a kind of fertilizer.

Just about every life-threatening disease you can name, from colon cancer and liver disease to hypertension and stroke, is strongly linked to obesity. Frequent fast-food consumption, with its excessive calories, makes it nearly impossible for the average person to maintain a healthy weight.

As a doctor, I see the painful effects of this every single day I go to work. Patients come to my office with arteries so clogged with fat deposits that blood can barely pass through them. Other patients have such severe diabetes that their bodies' own insulin can no longer transform food calories into energy. As a result, they live on daily injections, while excess blood sugar remains in their arteries, corroding them and blocking blood flow to tiny blood vessels. This frequently leads to blindness, gangrene, and amputation of their limbs. Still others harbor large cancerous tumors, which thrive in an environment of body fat. Body fat is also the home for C-reactive protein, an inflammatory marker that fans the fires of many dangerous diseases. Additionally, countless patients live with the constant pain and misery of arthritis, caused by overburdened joints worn out from bearing excess body weight over time.

Unless we make some significant changes, these health problems are only going to increase because American children are in worse shape than adults. When researchers examined the diets of teenagers at thirty-one city schools, they found that more than half ate fast food once or twice a week and took in an average of 2,192 calories a day. Those who ate fast food three or more times a week consumed an average of 2,752 calories. The normal adolescent body simply cannot process this overwhelming amount.

I used to blame the fast-food industry for all this. The excess sugar, fat, and calories they pack into their menu items are sure to trigger overweight and related diseases. Most processed foods are also loaded with artery-clogging trans-fatty acids and high-fructose corn syrup, both of which are literally toxic to our organs. I also got upset at school lunch programs that invite these franchises into the lunchroom because our schools' budgets have been slashed and they need the extra cash. And I would fume at the TV ads that bombard our kids with hyperclever pitches to make them crave these junky, fattening "treats."

But getting mad didn't do any good. So I got smarter.

No one wants the food police regulating what we can buy, sell, or eat. I realized that the fast-food industry will continue selling us these foods as long as we continue to buy them. And people will keep buying them until they make the diet-health connection for themselves. I wrote this book to help more people make this connection *before* they (or their kids) get hit with a serious health problem and to show people already hit with one how they can get better by eating better. Make no mistake—being overweight is an early warning sign of serious health trouble ahead. No amount of denial or nutritional ignorance will ever change that.

Fast food is here to stay. It's a permanent part of the North American landscape and lifestyle. It fits our schedule, it fits our budget, and we love the taste. So what's the solution? The only realistic answer to our weight woes is for you and people like you to get smarter, just like I did. That's what this book is all about.

In the pages ahead, you're going to learn how to lose weight and improve your health simply by making small, smart changes in your current eating habits—whether you're dining at home or ordering fast food. Yes, you really can lose weight and become healthier without giving up fast food!

Over the years, we've seen a bunch of weight-loss diets come and go: low-fat . . . low-carb . . . high-protein . . . vegetarian . . . plus many others. Yet today, Americans weigh more than ever. These approaches have not succeeded for three reasons. (1) They are difficult to understand and hard to follow. (2) Most require you to completely change your eating patterns. (3) Many have "rules" to obey and "taboo foods" to avoid. *The Fast-Food Diet* has none of these obstacles. It's easy to understand and it makes sense. It fits right into the way you currently eat. And there are no rules to follow, only a few tips and secrets that you can use whenever you like.

When I became a physician, I took an oath to help people. Writing this book is part of fulfilling that pledge. It's not enough to prescribe pills, recommend surgeries, and provide temporary relief of my patients' symptoms while ignoring the underlying cause of so many of these health problems. I'm talking about how and what we eat.

I specifically wrote this book to help nutritionally challenged North Americans. It's no coincidence that people who eat the most fast food have the least understanding of how these foods affect their weight and their health. Nor do they have the time or interest to explore the damage that excessive, indiscriminate consumption of these foods can do—until, perhaps, the damage has been done. So I'm passing this life-saving knowledge on to you—think of this as a nutritional house call.

Losing weight isn't rocket science. You don't need complicated theories, group therapy, or a gym membership. *The Fast Food Diet* will show you how to trim a few hundred calories from every meal without eating less food or depriving yourself of the flavors you've come to love. Those reduced calories will add up to pounds *lost* just as quickly and surely as those extra calories have been *increasing* your weight. As your weight and belly go down, your energy will increase. You'll look better and feel better about yourself. Best of all, your health will improve because how you eat is the single most important factor in avoiding today's plague of degenerative diseases. What you put in your mouth determines whether you'll live long or die young.

The greatest tragedy is that the medical conditions created by consuming so much are so unnecessary. If we ate just a few calories less at each meal and managed to be a bit more physically active every day, most of these health problems could be avoided or reversed. Experts have found that losing just 10 percent of our current body weight is all that it takes to turn many of these ills around and to increase our life span significantly.

Hippocrates, the first physician and the father of modern medicine, put it aptly more than two thousand years ago when he told his patients, "Let food be thy medicine." As a cardiologist and certified nutrition specialist (CNS), I can tell you that eating healthier food is going to be the salvation of tens of thousands—if not millions—of North Americans over the next decade. The demand for safer foods is not a fad; it's a trend. And it will grow even stronger as more people discover the profound truth that you are what you eat. In a perfect world, we'd all be much healthier and live a lot longer and better eating chemical-free organic food and less red meat, sugar, and fats. But ours, of course, is not a perfect world, so I'm offering a realistic compromise in this book that, if followed, will produce a significant improvement in your health and weight. Not everyone can afford to shop at Whole Foods or prepare healthy, home-cooked meals for their families every night. But anyone can easily learn how to make smarter choices, no matter where they eat—*even in fast-food restaurants*!

We are not being good role models for our children when we let ourselves get out of shape. Kids learn by imitation, and they eat and drink as we do. So save the lectures. Every good parent knows that children will follow what we *do*, not just what we say. We've got to lead them and love them by example.

Let this book be your road map to painless weight-loss success. Everything you'll need to know has been compressed and simplified into these few pages. Slip it into your purse when you go to lunch with your coworkers. Keep it in your car's glove compartment for smart advice while you're waiting in the drive-thru lane. Guided by the medically sound information in *The Fast Food Diet*, you'll always know what to avoid and what to substitute when making your food choices. In no time, you'll become a master at picking the best possible foods for health and weight loss in this fast-food world of ours.

Best of all, you'll be using brainpower instead of willpower to succeed. And that's really smart!

CHAPTER 1

The 80/20 Rule

Let's face it; some people just love fast food. We love the taste. We love the convenience. We love the price. And we can't get enough of it. Some of us have been eating it since we were kids. We literally cut our teeth on juicy cheeseburgers, crispy fries, and slushy milk shakes. I know I did. My first big job at age sixteen was managing a hamburger joint in my home town on Long Island, New York. I loved going to work because the food always smelled so good—and, as employees, we could eat all we wanted. (Back then, a burger with "the works" was fifteen cents!) Today, I'm a cardiologist and my job is fixing some of that artery damage I handed out in my teens.

But don't think this is another one of those fire-and-brimstone sermons about the evils of fast food. It isn't. Nutritionists and health experts have been condemning fast food for the last decade or so, and it hasn't made much of a difference.

America still leads the world in obesity, in heart attacks, in diabetes, and in cancer. It's time for a different approach and a more practical strategy.

So if you consider yourself a fast-food junkie—or you just can't imagine life without McDonald's, Pizza Hut, or Taco Bell (even though you probably know it's not doing your figure much good)—this book has some good news for you. It isn't going to scold or shame you. And it won't try to get you to forsake your fast-food habits. Instead, it's going to help you accomplish something revolutionary. Something that the health experts and weight-loss gurus say is impossible: to lose weight and improve your health while eating at the fast-food restaurants you've come to love.

Lose weight on fast food? Oh yes, it's possible.

We all know the story of Jared Fogel, the Indiana University student who once tipped the scales at 425 pounds. After trying (and failing at) numerous diets, he settled on a radical plan: two Subway submarine sandwiches a day—a six-inch turkey sub for lunch and a twelve-inch Veggie Delite for dinner. After a year on this diet, combined with daily exercise, he dropped 245 pounds. Since then, he's appeared on *Oprah* and *Larry King Live*. The Subway corporate offices report that people inspired by Fogel's example have lost a total of 160,000 pounds. Whoa!

And then there's Merab Morgan, the construction-worker mom from Raleigh, North Carolina, who ate only at McDonald's for ninety days and dropped 37 pounds in the process.

Impressed? The truth is, you can lose weight on almost *any* kind of food if you have iron willpower and a high threshold for boredom. Most of us have neither. If permanent weight-loss is what you're after, your diet needs variety and flavor so you'll stay interested. I'm willing to bet that, after a year of eating nothing but Subway sandwiches, Jared could barely stand to look at another sub if it weren't for the endorsement checks he is receiving.

I'm going to show you a much easier and more interesting way to lose weight. Most nutritionists call me a heretic because I tell people it's okay to eat fast food. It is—when you know a few tricks. Obviously, a steady diet of burgers and fries isn't going to help your waistline or your health. But if you know how and where to look, there's plenty of good stuff to be found in fast-food restaurants. This book will help you steer clear of the worst items on the menu—or, at least, help you limit your consumption without feeling deprived.

And that's the real key to long-term success: *knowledge*. We live and eat in the real world, so it's not realistic to expect people to completely abstain from fast food. No way are they going to. And that's fine—because there's absolutely nothing wrong with enjoying a Big Mac, a side of fries, or a shake once in a while.

I'm a big fan of the 80/20 Rule. I believe that if you're eating right about 80 percent of the time, it's okay to splurge the other 20 percent. The biggest reason most diet and exercise plans fail is that they're too rigid. They may work for a week or two, but sooner or later everyone gets tired of following the rules—and, rebels that we are, we break them. But the 80/20 Rule is one you can follow for life, because it gives you room to take a break. That's why the Fast-Food Diet succeeds.

Want proof? Medical studies show that people who are rigid and obsessive about losing weight—you know, the folks who count every carb, eat only special foods, never have dessert, gulp handfuls of vitamin pills and supplements, and so on— fail far more often than people who take a more balanced and flexible approach. The only thing being rigid is good for is making you feel bad about yourself when you slip. And that's a lousy way to succeed at anything.

The truth is, losing weight—or controlling how much you gain—is almost never just about willpower. How can it be? After all, you're dealing with hunger, one of the most powerful urges in life. No amount of willpower or self-discipline can overcome hunger for very long, because our very survival depends upon it.

Take it from a doctor who has been helping patients lose weight with this real-world strategy for decades: this approach really works. Little changes can make a big difference. And brainpower will win out over willpower every time.

In this book you'll learn how to eat smarter at home and in restaurants 80 percent of the time—whether they are of the drive-thru or sit-down variety. You'll see how to lose weight and become healthier, not by sacrificing or sweating, but simply by making wiser choices. Believe me, these small changes will quickly add up to big results. You're going to see your waistline shrink, your cholesterol fall, and your blood pressure plummet, while your energy level and your pride in your appearance start to soar.

And what about the other 20 percent of the time? Hey, that's your business. If you want to enjoy a little splurge, no problem. You won't be breaking any "rules" because, on *The Fast Food Diet*, there aren't any.

This easy-does-it strategy sure beats "eat less and exercise more"—plus a lot of other impossible-to-follow weight-loss schemes that have failed us over the years, such as low-fat diets, low-carb diets, high-protein diets, and many others.

Unlike most other nutritionists, I realize that condemning fast food in a culture like ours is a waste of time—it just doesn't work. Personally, I believe a *real* diet is far better than an ideal one.

For one thing, not all fast food is bad. There are quite a few menu items that are highly nutritious and modest in calories.

In the chapters ahead, I'll guide you to making smarter choices when you're dining out so you'll end up consuming fewer calories while feeling just as full and satisfied. You'll learn how to select the fast foods that are the most nutritious, are the best tasting, and will help you lose weight—even if you dine out three, four, or five times a week—or every day, for that matter!

Rest assured, your choices won't be limited to salads. Far from it. I'll point you to plenty of menu items that are off limits according to most nutritionists and weight-loss gurus— yet I'll show you how to enjoy them and still lose weight without feeling hungry an hour later. Besides, most fast-food salads are hardly weight-loss fare. You might be shocked to learn that a McDonald's salad with ranch dressing contains almost as many calories as a cheeseburger!

Are You a Candidate for a Heart Attack?

There's an easy way to tell. Once upon a time, doctors relied upon something called the body mass index (BMI) to determine who was at risk for heart disease. But these days, that's old-school. Scientists have just discovered a method that's more accurate—and much easier to calculate.

It's called the waist-to-hip ratio. You simply measure your waist and divide it by the measurement of your hips. If the number you get is higher than 0.85 in women or 0.9 in men, you're in the danger zone. The higher the waist-to-hip ratio, the higher your risk of heart attack. It's as simple as that.

And what if you find yourself over the cutoff point? The best way to lower your risk of a heart attack is to lose weight. That's what this book is all about.

The Fast-Food Diet is ultra-practical. It works by fitting into *your* lifestyle, instead of turning your daily schedule topsy-turvy. It shows you how to make clever little changes in eating habits you're already comfortable with, so you actually lose weight and improve your health without trying too hard. It's just what the doctor ordered because it makes the pleasure principle work *for* you.

As you're about to learn, it really is possible to lose weight on fast food. In fact, it's easier than you'd ever imagine. Take it from me: You can eat fast food several days of the week and still achieve sure and steady weight loss.

CHAPTER 2

Why Regular Diets Fail

Imagine, if you can, spending every waking moment of every single day in search of food, as our Stone Age ancestors did.

Your shrunken stomach would be constantly aching for something—*anything*—to eat. Your eyes would always search your surroundings for any edible morsel. Your children would cry and whimper from hunger. Frequently near-delirious from lack of nutrients, you'd eat roots, grubs, worms, wild bird eggs, leaves, berries, and even small dead animals you'd find on the trail.

Then, unexpectedly, you might come upon (or happen to kill) a larger animal. You and your clan would pounce on the carcass in a feeding frenzy that wouldn't end until only bare bones remained. When finished, you'd lick your greasy fingers clean, sigh, then belch. You'd be delighted by the rare occurrence of feeling your stomach being stuffed. Protein and fat would surge in your bloodstream. Glucose would course through your brain. This would be supreme pleasure—as close to ecstasy as it got in this primitive era. Stumbling in a food-induced stupor, you'd find a shady spot and slump against a tree for a rare break from your relentless foraging. Satisfied, you'd fall into a brief, deep sleep bordering on drunkenness.

Now, fast-forward twenty thousand years.

Today we no longer hunt for our food. Rather, we're surrounded by it. Supermarkets, restaurants, fast-food drive-thrus and convenience stores are everywhere, their shelves and refrigerated cases well stocked. In fact, food now hunts us, with sights and smells and ads seducing us to eat—and to do it often.

Nowadays, a complete meal—supplying the caloric equivalent of an entire day of hard work by our ancestors (a lucky day, that was)—is readily available for about a half-hour's pay, much less if you earn more than the minimum wage.

You're Genetically Programmed to Eat More and Eat Rich

Back in the early days of human development, our ancestors expended up to 1,500 calories or more per day in search of food. Often, the energy they spent in their daily quest *exceeded* the calories they found. Deficit eating was the rule of the day. Needless to say, there were no overweight or obese people. On those rare occasions when our ancestors happened upon a large supply of food, they gorged themselves until they couldn't eat another bite. They did this for two reasons. First, they were ravenous with hunger. But more important, they instinctively knew they had to store as many calories as possible to get them through the lean days and weeks ahead. When the body misses a meal, it actually holds on to its fat reserves and burns calories at a slower-than-normal rate. This is why dieting isn't a very successful way to lose weight—because eating less causes the body to hoard its fat.

Why am I telling you all this? I want you to understand that the primary reason we are so overweight today is *not* our supposed lack of willpower or self-discipline. Instead, it is genetic programming that has evolved the human body into a fat-storage machine designed for survival. Let me explain.

Calories are a measure of the energy contained in our food. Our bodies are able to process only about 600 to 900 calories per meal. Anything above this amount is immediately converted into fat and stored in case we aren't able to eat again anytime soon. When times are lean, our bodies naturally slow the rate at which those stored fat calories are burned, rationing them until we need a sudden burst of energy, say for running after (or away from) a wild animal.

This mechanism served humankind remarkably well during the prehistoric days of hunting and gathering, but today it's an enemy within us when it comes to maintaining a healthy weight. In the industrialized parts of the world, every meal is a feast without the threat of famine. The result is that we store more and more energy in the form of body fat around our hips, thighs, bellies, necks, and jowls that we will never burn off unless we choose to be physically active.

In contrast to third world populations, people in developed countries are dying from the results of *too much* food. Overconsumption of calories is causing a variety of degenerative diseases that are cutting years off our lives and making middle and old age uncomfortable, if not downright miserable.

It's *What* You Eat, Not How Much

We are genetically programmed to eat until the sensation of "fullness" sets in—a complex response involving blood sugar levels, brain chemicals, and other biological factors, aided by tiny "stretch receptors" in the stomach that signal the brain when its capacity has been reached. The human stomach is a pouch about the size of a clenched fist. Most people assume it to be larger, but normally it isn't. However, the stomach will stretch in size if we continually cram it with food. When this happens, the stomach requires ever-increasing amounts of food to trigger the stretch receptors that signal fullness. But this overeating isn't the main reason we become overweight, because it isn't *how much* food we pack into our stomachs that causes the problem, but rather the *kind* of food. Calories, not the volume, are the real culprit. This is an important distinction, and understanding it is the single most important key to controlling your weight, or slimming down.

Ounce for ounce, modern processed foods contain far more calories than anything found in nature. They are loaded with extra fat, which contains more than twice as many calories per gram as carbohydrates and protein. Many commercial foods also contain added sweeteners in the form of high-fructose corn syrup, a highly concentrated source of calories. We also eat loads of refined, calorie-dense carbohydrates such as breads, cookies, cakes, crackers, and candies, to name just a few of the popular foods that pack an enormous amount of calories into a few bites.

One of the most extreme examples of these calorie-concentrated foods is what we have come to call fast food—a greasy hamburger topped with cheese, slathered with mayonnaise-based sauce, and sandwiched between a big bread bun. This is a meal unto itself; but it is frequently served with a side of deep-fat-fried french fries and a soft drink that can contain the equivalent of 40 teaspoons of sugar.

By the time your stomach signals it is full from the physical volume of one of these calorie-intense meals, you could have easily consumed 1,200 calories or more. This is nearly twice as many calories as the body can put to immediate use, so the excess is converted into fat and stored away in your fat cells. Just one meal like this contains nearly all the calories needed by the average female, whose intake shouldn't exceed 1,800 calories per day if she doesn't want to gain weight.

Add to this a breakfast, a sit-down dinner, a few snacks, and another soft drink or two or three, and it's easy to see the enormous impact that a simple fast-food lunch can have on your weight and, ultimately, your health.

So here we are, surrounded by an unprecedented abundance of food that is more concentrated in calories than anything humans have ever known. To make matters worse, we are conditioned to eat three meals a day. "Three squares a day" was a necessity back in the days when our forefathers were hard-working farm families. Back then, the average man and woman labored from sunrise to sunset—the equivalent of running ten miles a day—requiring as many as 5,000 calories a day.

Our Sedentary Lifestyle

Today, we perform much less physical labor, but the habit of eating three daily meals prevails. Our bellies have grown accustomed to feeling full; in fact, many of us feel a vague "emptiness" when they are not. Cars carry us everywhere, making it easy to miss the physical activity necessary to burn these calories. Many of you who are my age (fifty-nine) can recall walking to school as a child. Of course, that's not the case today. And before the advent of television, kids went outdoors to play baseball, football, tag, and to exhaust themselves on the public playground. Now, our kids mostly play video games, watch TV, and are chauffeured everywhere by parents and school buses.

Adults are in a similar bind. Work is more intellectual than manual, and what little leisure time we have is spent recovering from the day's stress on the couch, usually with an ample supply of calorie-packed snack foods. Is it any wonder we are in such poor shape?

Health officials first announced that we had a problem back in the early 1980s. Reacting to the threat of rising rates of obesity, heart disease, and other weight-related conditions, people began jogging, running, biking, swimming, jumping rope, and doing step aerobics. All sorts of hamster-wheel exercise devices were invented. People joined gyms, pumped weights, and became martial artists, rock climbers, kayakers, marathoners, jazz dancers—anything to burn fat and build muscle. America was in the grip of a fitness-and-dieting craze that turned people into fanatics and left them feeling hungry and exhausted. Hundreds of thousands of people today are still running themselves ragged in the pursuit of losing weight.

At any given moment—like right now—50 percent of all adults in this country are involved in some type of effort to lose weight. Some are dieting (formally known as *calorie restriction*, a fancy way of saying "eating less food"). Some are exercising their buns off. Some have joined national weight-loss organizations. Some drink exotic beverages or pop pills and supplements that speed up their metabolism, or munch low-calorie energy bars in place of regular meals.

This, of course, makes the diet industry a huge industry. By 2008, it will be worth $61 billion. Why so big? Because there is a lot of repeat business in the weight-loss industry. People hop from fad to fad because so few of these approaches succeed. Research from as far back as the 1950s has found that about 95 percent of all diets fail.

While the official failure rate for dieting may not surprise you, this will: Over the past few decades, the American public has been part of a massive experiment. Doctors and self-proclaimed weight-loss experts have been plying us with weight-loss theories that have no real scientific backing. That includes the two most popular crazes of recent times, the low-fat diet and the low-carb diet. Each deserves close scrutiny because millions of people in this country were (and still are) devotees.

What's Wrong about the Low-Fat Craze

The low-fat diet got started in the 1970s. Though this approach was never scientifically proven, it seemed to make sense. Since fat has twice as many calories as carbohydrates or protein, it seemed logical that consuming fatty foods—including fried foods, red meat, cheese, and other dairy products—was the fast lane to weight gain. Low-fat eating became the rage, and an entirely new category of reduced-fat foods filled supermarket shelves. We had no-fat cookies, fat-free ice creams, low-fat pastries, nonfat milk and cheeses, and on and on. Every food manufacturer was eager to capitalize on this new diet craze.

But a curious thing happened. After fifteen years of eating less fat, scientists discovered that Americans hadn't slimmed down at all. In fact, we had grown progressively fatter. During the years when fat consumption was dropping, the weight of the average American adult *increased* by about 10 pounds. Why? Because Americans, believing that low-fat foods would help them lose weight, ate more of them. It wasn't unusual in those days for an individual to consume an entire box of low-fat cookies in one sitting.

As a cardiologist, I bought into the low-fat theory too. Meats and other fat sources disappeared from our dining room table and our cupboards began to fill with low-fat "light" pasta meals and no-fat salad dressings. I even fed our Norwegian elkhound Charlie the same "healthy" food we were eating. Needless to say, while we loved the carbohydrate foods and snacks that filled our bellies, my wife and I were packing on the pounds—and so was our dog! After the final verdict on low-fat came out, I had to rewrite the guidelines in my book, *Optimum Health*, for a revised edition.

"Carbo-mania"

Like everyone else, we were eating less fat, but we were actually taking in more calories from the carbohydrates in these foods than if we had eaten the full-fat versions. So guess what became the next "problem" food group for overweight people? In the late 1980s, carbohydrates became the new dietary demon, ushering in a new era of low-carb eating. Led by Dr. Robert Atkins, America's low-carb guru, our nation embarked on a diet craze that bordered on compulsion. Protein became the new weight-loss "miracle" food, and eating carbohydrate foods such as bread, pasta, white rice, grains, and sugar was tantamount to dietary mortal sin.

Dr. Atkins encouraged his followers to eat protein—and lots of it—at every meal. People were having eggs, bacon, and sausage for breakfast, while skipping the fruit, juice, toast, and breakfast cereals. Lunch was a bun-less hamburger, a hunk of cheese, and a tall glass of milk. Dinners consisted of steaks, chops (or both), and maybe a small side of broccoli or a salad with blue cheese or ranch dressing. Restaurants obliged by offering heaps of meat and cutting back on the potatoes.

Even though the medical community soundly criticized the diet as being dangerous to cardiovascular health because of its high saturated fat content (as well as encouraging bone loss and overburdening the kidneys with excessive protein), low-carb eating spread like wildfire from coast to coast. Given permission to eat all the rich, savory meat and cheese they wanted as a way to lose weight, millions of people jumped on the bandwagon. The food industry wasted no time hopping on board too, creating entire lines of low-carb foods, many of which were endorsed by the suddenly wealthy Atkins corporation. The main attraction, of course, was that people were free to eat the once-forbidden fatty foods they've always loved. As one medical critic put it: "People always love to hear good news about their bad habits."

In reality, high-protein, low-carb diets like Atkins's actually do work—at least in the beginning. When the body runs out of stored carbohydrates, it begins burning fat for energy. It wasn't unusual for folks on Atkins-type diets to lose 5, 10, even 20 pounds during the first month or so. Word quickly spread, and the popularity of the low-carb diet grew.

Unfortunately, this impressive weight loss didn't continue; it invariably ceased within a few months. Doctors later discovered why. The Atkins diet forces the body into an abnormal state called *ketosis*, where potentially toxic *ketones* are created in the tissues. When the body creates ketones, they need to be eliminated, causing people on these diets to urinate a lot. This initial weight loss was little more than water. The body's fat reserves were barely being touched.

Actually, just the opposite was occurring: body fat was increasing. That's because eating excessive amounts of protein raises the amount of insulin in the bloodstream. And one of insulin's jobs is to convert excess calories, whether they come from protein or carbohydrates, into body fat. When people finally saw the long-term effect that the various low-carb diets were producing, they dropped them like hot potatoes.

A study conducted by Tufts University Medical School found that 22 percent of people on either low-carb or low-fat diets abandoned them after two months. After a year, the dropout rate was 50 percent.

The Happy Medium

Around the time that the low-fat diet was being abandoned and the low-carb craze was taking off, a young scientist named Dr. Barry Sears developed a weight-loss approach that was very different from either of these extremes, called the Zone Diet. Dr. Sears argued that it was too simple-minded to blame either fats or carbohydrates for our weight woes. The real problem, he said, was the *kind* of fats and carbohydrates we were eating. He was one of the first to state that there are good and bad fats, as well as good and bad carbs.

I want to tip my hat to Dr. Barry Sears, whose pioneering research and scientific insights recognized the inherent flaws in both the low-fat fad and the low-carb craze early on. His groundbreaking book, *The Zone*, which describes one of the most sane, sensible, and balanced diets ever conceived, has helped countless thousands of people to lose weight and improve their health. His "40-30-30" dietary recommendation (that our diets should be about 40 percent low-glycemic-index carbohydrates, 30 percent protein, and 30 percent fats) has stood the test of time and scientific scrutiny. We all owe him a debt of gratitude.

Carbohydrates are natural sugars that are present in just about all foods, with the exception of animal products, oils, and other fats. Sears described "good carbs" as carbohydrates in their whole, natural state. Examples are fresh fruits, vegetables, and whole grains. Because these foods are not refined (meaning their fiber content has not been reduced or removed), they are bulkier, contain fewer calories by volume, and are digested more slowly. Hence, the stomach becomes filled with a greater volume of food but fewer calories. Since this feeling of fullness lasts longer, it takes longer before you are hungry again. The result? You eat less frequently and therefore lose weight.

Good Carbs, Bad Carbs

Refined carbs are the dietary black sheep of the carbohydrate family. They've had their bulk and fiber removed so they are a more concentrated form of calories. Because their volume has been diminished by milling, one can eat more of them before the stomach registers full. That's just one reason they are so fattening.

A bigger problem results when many of these refined carbs are combined with other high-calorie ingredients. When white flour, a refined grain that has had its fiber milled away, is mixed with eggs, oil, milk, and a little sweetener—as is usually done to make white bread, pastries, or other baked goods—the calorie content jumps, but its volume increases only slightly. These "white carbs" trigger an instant spike in blood sugar (glucose) levels. When the body senses the spike, it orders the pancreas to manufacture more insulin for release into the bloodstream. There insulin helps break down the glucose into fuel for our brain cells and muscles, but when faced with a surplus, the excess sugar is swiftly metabolized into fat and stored in our fat cells. This mechanism was crucial for our ancestors' survival (a hedge against a rainy day when food was scarce) but it spells double trouble these days. Refined carbohydrates make it easy for your body to pack on the weight more quickly, while making it more difficult to lose.

As if that weren't bad enough, there's an even darker side to the rush of insulin that happens when your blood sugar spikes. Doctors have found that it promotes inflammation in the body, setting the stage for artery disease, heart attack, Alzheimer's, even cancer, while making inflammatory conditions such as arthritis hurt more. *As a cardiologist, I must warn you that the single most inflammatory agent in the body that causes coronary artery disease is the excess insulin in the bloodstream caused by refined carbohydrates.*

Add to this the diabetes connection. Constantly asking the body to produce insulin weakens its effect (called insulin resistance) and exhausts the cells in the pancreas that produce it. This causes adult-onset, or Type 2, diabetes. Diabetes is *the* health crisis of the twenty-first century. If you get it, diabetes will shorten your life by an average of ten years. You'll be forced to inject yourself with insulin up to four times a day. Your risk of heart attack and stroke will skyrocket. On top of that, diabetes is the leading cause of blindness, and it increases your risk of having your legs amputated by fifteen times. The disease currently affects 150 million people worldwide and causes five million deaths a year. The World Health Organization (WHO) predicts those numbers will double in twenty years, causing the first reduction in life expectancy in two hundred years. The massive amount of sugar and refined carbohydrates in the modern diet are the main reason. Believe me, this is a truly horrible disease, one you want to avoid by all means. And the best way is to limit your intake of refined carbohydrates.

But not all carbs lead to diabetes and weight gain. Dr. Sears helped define the difference between a good carb and a bad carb by popularizing the Glycemic Index (see appendix A on page 221). This chart ranks how quickly (or slowly) a carbohydrate releases its sugar into the bloodstream. The lower a food's Glycemic Index, the more slowly it releases its sugars, and the less it raises blood glucose after meals. Sears went on to define the Glycemic Load—a measure of total daily consumption of carbs that affect blood sugar levels—as being the single most important factor in predicting insulin release. The GI chart lists the best foods for weight loss toward the top of this chart because they trigger the least insulin release. This is extremely valuable information to know.

Limiting your consumption of refined carbohydrates (high GI) is one of the most important things you can do to lose weight and improve your health. That's because the body's storage capacity for surplus carbohydrates is quite limited. Only about 300 to 400 grams (about 12 ounces) can be stored in your muscles, and 60 to 90 grams (2 to 3 ounces) can be contained in your liver. Once this storage capacity is reached, any additional carbohydrates you consume that aren't used as fuel by your metabolism are immediately converted into fat and stored in your fat cells, especially around your abdomen and hips.

Just so you know, the typical fast-food meal contains an astonishing amount of refined carbohydrates. If you order a burger, fries, and shake, you could easily gulp down more than 150 grams (about 5½ ounces) of refined carbohydrates. To put this in perspective, the average adult male requires about 2,000 calories per day, with no more that 40 percent of those calories coming from carbohydrates (approximately 200 grams, or about 7 ounces). This one fast-food meal contains nearly 80 percent of the recommended carb intake for the entire day!

Now you understand why you've got to be knowledgeable about what you order in your favorite fast-food restaurant. If you aren't careful, those calories can show up around your waistline and make you a candidate for diabetes very quickly.

Dietary Fats: The Good, the Bad, and the Ugly

As with carbohydrates, not all fats are bad, either. Dr. Sears correctly pointed out that some fats are actually essential for good health. It's important to recognize a good fat and a bad one. The biggest public enemies in the fat world, according to Dr. Sears and most scientists today, are saturated fats and trans fats. Why are they so bad? For one thing, they cause inflammation in the body. But even worse, they cause the body to produce harmful compounds called *eicosanoids*, hormone-like substances that increase blood pressure and promote blood clotting (a prescription for stroke), and trigger inflammation in the arteries (a major cause of heart attack). To add insult to injury, eicosanoids make it difficult for the body to burn stored fat, promoting weight gain.

Unfortunately, many fast-food menu items contain massive amounts of saturated fat and trans fat. These fats not only pack *twice* the amount of calories as protein and carbs, but they also trigger an onslaught of free-radical molecules that damage the body's cells and accelerate the aging process. That's why it's so important to think twice before you order—and learn how to eat healthier.

The good guys of the fat world are monounsaturated fats, which predominate in olive oil. They actually reduce inflammation and lower the risk of heart disease by not eliciting the insulin response and making it easier for your body to burn off its fat reserves. Whenever possible, you should substitute olive oil for any other fat or oil you are offered. One final point: you have to eat fat in order to lose it. Without sufficient fat intake, your metabolism can't work properly. I'll tell you more about these beneficial fats later on.

Is it really possible to lose weight by eating fat? Absolutely. In a landmark study conducted almost fifty years ago, people on a low-calorie diet, *with 90 percent of the calories coming from fat*, actually lost weight. When the same people switched to a diet consisting of the same number of calories coming from 90 percent carbohydrates, they failed to lose a pound. Just keep in mind that all fats, good or bad, have the same number of calories (9 per gram) so you never want to overdo it—especially at salad bars, where this is easy to do. In other words, don't overdo it on the olive oil.

If all this talk about good and bad fats and carbohydrates is making your eyes glaze over, don't worry. The next few chapters make it easy for you by guiding you to the best fast-food menu choices and steering you away from the worst. Forget about rules and absolutes. Just remember that small, easy changes like those you'll discover in this book (and more on our free Web site at www.thefastfooddiet.com) are what really make the difference. For instance, if you burn about 250 calories with a brisk walk and trim about 250 calories a day from your diet (the amount in a small order of Wendy's fries), this alone would add up to about half a pound of weight loss a week. You'd weigh 25 pounds less in a year's time!

My message to you is: Take heart. The verdict from the world's largest database of people who have lost an average of 60 pounds and kept it off for an average of 10 years proves that losing weight permanently is possible. *But not by dieting*. Read on.

CHAPTER 3

The Secrets of Easy Weight-Loss Success

Most people only need to lose about 10 percent of their body weight to prevent or reverse serious health problems. And as you'll learn in the chapters ahead, this is easy to accomplish. Losing weight isn't complex or even difficult. You don't even have to give up your favorite restaurants or fast-food drive-thrus to succeed.

Of course, we all know people who have lost weight on the latest trendy diet. While it's tempting to think that these folks have more willpower than we do or know some magical secret we don't, *the real secret is that there isn't any mystery to slimming down*. It's not rocket science; it's just simple math: if you eat more calories than you burn, your body will gain weight. If your daily intake of calories pretty much equals what you burn, your weight will remain stable. If you eat fewer calories or burn more than your body needs to maintain itself, you'll lose weight. There are no gimmicks, shortcuts, or loopholes around this fundamental law of nature.

Do the Math

Your body will lose 1 pound for every 3,500 calories you shave from your diet. The most painless way to accomplish this is by *simply eating 500 fewer calories a day*—or burning off that many—or some combination of both. It doesn't matter whether those calories come from home cooking, restaurant meals, or fast food. Forgo or burn a mere 500 extra calories every day and you'll shed the weight. Sounds easy? It is. To prove it, here are some tips to illustrate just how easy losing weight this way can be:

Keep your pantry and fridge well stocked

Most weight-loss attempts fail because of poor planning. If your refrigerator and pantry lack a variety of healthful, low-calorie foods, you'll grab whatever is handy when you get hungry. If you buy chips, candy, ice cream, and other fattening treats when you shop, that's what you'll eat when your blood sugar dips and makes you hungry. So if you shop a little smarter, you'll naturally eat the good stuff when you arrive home as hungry as a bear.

Eat five times a day

Most people trying to lose weight don't eat breakfast. Many skip lunch as well. So by 5 p.m. they're ravenous and often consume more calories at dinner than they would if they ate three sensible meals a day. They've also thrown their bodies into fat-hoarding mode by eating a giant meal. Eating three meals a day and snacking in between controls your hunger and prevents your blood sugar levels from dipping too low, which makes you want to eat, eat, eat.

Dinner is the largest meal of the day for most Americans. Unfortunately, this works against weight loss. In laboratory studies, animals who consumed most of their calories at night gained more weight than those taking in an equal number of calories throughout the day. Reason? The body's secretion of insulin peaks in the evening and extra insulin ensures that more of the calories you eat will be stored as fat. You'll lose weight more easily if you eat more of your calories at breakfast and lunch and fewer at dinner.

Eat lean protein with every meal

Protein curbs hunger more effectively than fat or carbohydrates. If you want to test this yourself, have a bagel for breakfast, then clock how long it takes before you're feeling hungry again. The next morning, eat that same bagel slathered with a tablespoon or two of peanut butter. You'll see that this extra protein will keep you full for at least an additional two hours.

Try to eat at least 15 to 20 grams of protein with every meal—and more is even better. You'll get that much from one egg or a bowl of oatmeal for breakfast, a Sonic burger for lunch, and one of Wendy's Mandarin Chicken Salads for supper. When you find yourself hungry an hour or two after eating, it means you probably need to up the amount of protein in your meals.

Get enough good fat

Many so-called experts advise you to reduce the fat in your diet. But as you'll see in the next chapter, between 25 and 30 percent of your daily calories should come from fat—yet always in the form of fish, nuts, olive oil, or other sources of healthful fats. Adequate amounts of fat cause your metabolism to operate more efficiently, burning calories instead of storing them. As a bonus, it also promotes the absorption of fat-soluble nutrients such as vitamin D, vitamin K, and coenzyme Q_{10}.

Don't depend on "white" carbohydrates

This means white rice, pasta, white bread, and other starchy foods. There's nothing wrong with eating these foods on occasion. And I'm not suggesting you peel the white bun off a burger and toss it in the trash, but white carbohydrates raise your blood sugar almost as fast as pure sugar does. After this initial spike, massive amounts of insulin are released into the bloodstream to quickly move the blood sugar (glucose) into your muscles, your liver, and your brain. Once the blood sugar is removed, you not only feel hungry again but will crave more carbohydrates. Additionally, refined white carbs encourage your metabolism to turn excess calories into fat and store them in your fat cells. Eating these foods in the evening when insulin is higher almost guarantees weight gain.

If you find that your energy consistently dips after eating, or you frequently become sleepy, it's usually because you've had too many of this type of carbs. To lose weight and have a steady supply of energy (instead of the roller-coaster kind), eat more unrefined foods such as brown rice, beans, legumes, whole grains, and vegetables. (Sorry, french fries don't count.)

Take it home

This one simple tip could save you several hundred calories per meal. Studies reveal that people tend to eat as much as 40 percent more when they dine out. You actually eat less by having a take-out meal and bringing it home. In addition, eating fast food at home gives you the option of serving up healthier side dishes along with the main course, such as salads or steamed vegetables.

Order dressing on the side

This might sound trivial, but it's often the condiments and restaurant side orders, especially salad dressing, that can really pack on extra pounds. Consider a salad topped with Newman's Own Ranch Dressing offered at McDonald's. The dressing alone has 170 calories. Switching to Newman's Own Low-Fat Balsamic Vinaigrette drops the calorie count down to 40. Even better, order it on the side and drizzle on only a small amount.

Eat slowly—and mindfully

A lot of the calories we consume are "mindless" calories. These are the result of automatic, hand-to-mouth feeding when we're occupied with other things, like snacking in front of the TV or wolfing down calories at a bar. Eating on the run—when your stomach has no time to catch up with your brain—almost guarantees that you'll take in more calories than you would if you sat down and really enjoyed your food.

Americans gobble their meals far more quickly than people in France, Italy, or other Mediterranean countries. Rapid eating is a sure-fire way to take in excess calories. Here's why: once your stomach's stretch receptors sense that it is close to being full, they send a signal to your brain to stop eating. Unfortunately, this signal can take as long as twenty minutes to get there. So people who eat quickly tend to consume a lot of extra calories before their brains get the message. Here's how to avoid this:

■ Keep your hunger under control by eating frequently, say every two or three hours. This will prevent you from becoming so famished that you practically inhale your food when it's set in front of you.

- Take smaller bites and chew slowly. Appreciate the aroma, texture, and flavors, rather than gulping down your food.

- Eat at the table, not at the kitchen counter. This will help you relax, slow down, and appreciate the food's flavors and aromas.

- Get in the habit of putting smaller amounts of food on your plate and on your fork. Don't overload, either.

- Set down your fork between bites. Pick it up again after you've chewed and swallowed your food. Americans have a habit of filling their fork for a second bite before they've finished the first. Food-in-hand quickly becomes food-in-mouth.

Take smaller portions

Forget those hard-to-remember rules about portion sizes. They don't work, because everyone requires different amounts of food. However, taking a little less than you think you want generally works. Studies show that people typically overestimate the amount of food they need—but once it's on their plate they eat it, even if they've already had enough.

Plan on seconds

That's right, I said "seconds." This clever trick works in two ways. First, you can take a little less with your first helping without feeling like you're dieting. Second, putting some time between a first and second helping gives your brain time to receive your stomach's "I'm full" signal. Because we've been so conditioned since childhood to clean our plates and not waste food, we usually eat what's in front of us even if we're not really hungry. A smaller second serving will help you steer clear of these extra calories. This tip helps shrink the size of your stomach without making you feel deprived. Your stomach actually stretches when you indulge yourself with heaping first servings on a regular basis. This trains it to need larger amounts of food to become satisfied. Cutting down your serving sizes reverses the process, actually reducing the size of your stomach and triggering chemical reactions in your brain that lessen your body's demand for food.

Why Soft Drinks Are So Fattening

Carbonated soft drinks are the single biggest source of calories in the North American diet, accounting for about 7 percent of our daily calories. According to the Center for Science in the Public Interest, teenagers get 13 percent of their calories from soft drinks. The average American drinks upward of 50 gallons of soft drinks annually!

Apart from their water content, soft drinks are mainly refined sugar. Teens suck down the equivalent of 15 teaspoons of refined sugar daily in sodas. That's about the top end of the carbohydrate limit that experts recommend for all foods combined in a day!

Soft drinks have been named as one of the leading causes of overweight and obesity—along with Type 2 diabetes and other weight-related illnesses. They contain high-fructose corn syrup (HFCS), which is toxic to the body, in particular the liver. HFCS also causes profound fat accumulation and weight gain. This inexpensive sweetener is dumped into soft drinks and is added to literally thousands of foods, from cookies and jams to supersized muffins.

It's not merely the extra calories that make it such a nutritional nightmare. There's evidence that high-fructose corn syrup acts differently in the body than regular sugar and may increase the risk of serious diseases. HFCS also causes a rise in triglycerides, the blood fats that have been linked to heart disease. Animal studies indicate that a high-fructose diet can trigger insulin resistance and excess levels of insulin. Even without these dangers, the extra calories alone are a good enough reason to avoid it.

In 1970, the average adult ate about half a pound of HFCS a year. Now that's risen to about 70 pounds! Kids—with smaller bodies and a big thirst for sweets—chug down even more. It's not only the sugar that makes sodas a problem, but also what they replace in kids' diets. Children used to drink a lot more milk than soda. In the mid-1990s, the balance turned and children were drinking twice as much soda as milk. At the same time, they began getting lower amounts of vitamins and minerals in their diet.

Want to lose weight without trying? Give up (or cut back) the soft drinks. At 140 calories per 12-ounce serving, you could easily lose half a pound a week (or more) by simply switching to water, ice tea, or carbonated seltzer from the soft drink fountain with just a dash of Sprite, 7-Up, or lemonade added for flavor. Here are some other tips:

- Read food labels and limit your consumption of any beverages or foods that list HFCS as one of the first three or four ingredients.

- Since corn syrup is the main ingredient in sodas, cutting back on them will make losing weight much easier. Try to substitute seltzer or sparkling water with a squeeze of lemon every once in a while (or more often, if you can).

- Go for smaller drink sizes. Those Big Gulp cups are belly-busters—and a sure path to diabetes. If you must have bigger sized drinks, fill a Big Gulp cup halfway with club soda or seltzer from the soda fountain and the other half with your favorite soft drink. You'll be cutting your calories by 50 percent.

Go for the smaller sips

At most fast-food chains, it doesn't seem to make economic sense to get the smaller drinks, because the bigger sizes cost just a few cents more. Marketers plan it this way to encourage you to supersize your food and drinks. But the calorie difference can be significant. A large, 32-ounce cola contains about 310 calories. If you switch to the 16-ounce size instead, you'll reduce the number of calories by half. (Remember: To lose a pound a week—or 50 pounds a year—you only need to reduce your daily calorie intake by 500 calories. This one painless switch gets you one-third of the way there!) Even better: You can eliminate soda calories entirely by drinking water or

Quick Cuts

Take a hypothetical hamburger meal at any fast-food restaurant. By the time you've totaled up the meat patty (500 calories, at least), the bun (about 160 calories), the "special sauce" (easily 150 calories), a big order of fries (about 800 calories), and an average cola (about 170 calories), you've swallowed in excess of 1,600 calories. That's almost the total calorie need for a 120-pound woman for the entire day! It's a whopping amount, but you're probably getting even more in the form of condiments (one tablespoon of mayo adds about 100 calories) and other add-ons.

So try this weight-loss trick: Go to the same restaurant, have grilled chicken instead of the beef patty, eliminate (or reduce) the condiments, order a club soda with lemon, and substitute a baked potato (without butter or sour cream topping) for the fries. You'll easily cut the calorie load by half while feeling just as full. You'll also be getting a lot less fat—good for your heart as well as your hips.

seltzer with lemon. If you drop a 300-plus calorie soda from your diet five times a week, you'll lose nearly a half a pound a week. Or you won't gain it. If you must have an occasional soda, dilute it with seltzer or soda water and you'll save a bunch of calories.

Downsize, don't supersize

At most restaurants, a single serving usually provides enough fat and calories for two daily meals. It's not a bad idea to get in the habit of ordering "half sizes" from the menu. Or you can order a child's meal and see if that satisfies you, because this is usually the correct amount of food. When we dine out, my wife and I often order one entrée and share it. With soup and salad, that's plenty! Or, since it's often cheaper (relatively speaking) to get the larger portions, go ahead and order the standard serving and take half home for later.

Fear the Fries

Without a doubt, fast-food french fries pose the worst danger to your weight and health. Nearly everyone loves them—even people who aren't fast-food junkies. Yet french fries are often soaked with trans fats, chemically altered oils that are an even greater risk for heart disease than saturated fats like butter and lard. French fries are also high in *acrylamide*, a chemical that forms in starchy foods like potatoes when they're cooked in very hot fat and is known to cause cancer in laboratory animals. And we haven't even talked about the excessive salt sprinkled on them.

What should you do? No one wants the food police ordering them to hand over their fries. But you don't want to keel over from a stroke or heart attack either, do you? So try this for compromise. If you have an irresistible craving for fries, order the small size and eat them s-l-o-w-l-y. Like one at a time. Enjoy every bite . . . and leave a few for a friend. Feeling better? Good. Because, in all honesty, you've reached your fry limit. This is one fast food you *can't* have every week if you want to lose weight—or keep your blood fats in the healthy zone. Besides the deadly trans fats and cancer-causing acrylamide, french fries are loaded with calories. A typical small order packs between 200 and 300 of them. You'd have to walk between two and three miles to burn them off—and even then your arteries would still be stuck with the extra-fatty load.

How Hungry Are You *Really*?

While a few of the fast food chains have cut back on their portions, "supersize" still sells in America. McDonald's current Quarter Pounder, the original supersize burger, seems almost dainty today at a mere 700 calories. By contrast, the Double Whopper at Burger King approaches 1,000 calories. That's half the calories the average person needs for an entire day!

Before you order: Ask yourself if your appetite really demands that much chow. A little forethought and knowledge will really help. Consider this:

- The McDonald's Quarter Pounder with cheese, a 16-ounce soda, and an order of large fries contain 1,166 calories.
- The McDonald's regular hamburger with small fries and a 16-ounce club soda weighs in at 481 calories.

If you did nothing else in your weight-loss efforts but switch to the second, smaller meal, you'd save over 3,400 calories a week. With this one simple change, you'd lose one pound a week! That's 50 pounds a year! How would you like to lose 50 pounds without giving up fast food? Keep reading to see how.

Escape the Salt Mine!

By now most of us know that a high-salt diet is a major risk factor for hypertension, stroke, and heart attack. And it increases your weight. The body has a mechanism for keeping the salt level in the blood and tissues constant. If you eat a lot of salt, the body dilutes the blood and tissue fluids by retaining more water. But did you realize that the average American consumes twenty to thirty times more salt than his or her body needs? And that's if you never pick up the salt shaker.

Nearly 80 percent of our daily salt intake comes from hidden sources like prepared foods, including fast food. Consider the "healthy" McDonald's McVeggie sandwich. It contains 1,200 milligrams of salt, 80 percent of the *upper* recommended daily limit. McDonald's is hardly alone. You can easily get a day's worth of salt (or more) in a single meal at virtually any restaurant chain. It's almost impossible to avoid salt when you eat out.

You can help lower your salt intake by choosing fish instead of a burger or chicken. For example, a McDonald's filet of fish has 640 mg. of sodium versus 1,140 mg for a Double Cheeseburger and 1,210 mg for a Premium Grilled Chicken Classic. A baked potato (one of nature's best sources of heart-healthy potassium) is much better for you than french fries. More realistically, since most restaurant food is awash in salt, you should plan on cutting back on processed, packaged, and other salt-rich foods when you're eating at home, where you can control the ingredients. If you are salt-sensitive or have blood pressure problems, a good general rule for healthy eating is this: If you eat fast food today, don't eat any food that's packaged in a can or box tomorrow.

Avoid "Addictive" Foods

Just about everyone who struggles with their weight has a few "problem foods." By this I mean snacks or treats that are so seductive and tantalizing that giving them up would take almost superhuman strength.

One of nature's ironies is that these foods are *never* good for you. They're things like crackers and chips. Greasy fast-food burgers and fries. Wedges of cheese. Chocolate and ice cream. The specific foods hardly matter; they're different for everyone. But we all know which ones are a problem for us individually—and being free from the spell they cast over us would sure help us budge those stubborn pounds.

Why don't we just quit eating them? For the same reason that smokers have such a hard time quitting or drug addicts keep going back for more. The truth is, certain foods affect the brain the same way heroin and nicotine do. They produce neurochemical changes that are addictive. That's why willpower alone is never enough to erase their power over us —and why so many people say things like, "I know I have to quit eating [fill in the blank], but I just can't."

In his fascinating book *Breaking the Food Seduction*, Neal Barnard, M.D., reports on a study in which a group of choco-holics was given a drug called *naloxone*, which prevents narcotics from affecting the brain. After taking the drug, the volunteers were offered a tray filled with M&M's and other chocolate snacks. Normally, these chocolate-cravers would have pounced on the candy. But after taking the drug, they had no interest. Why? Because chocolate affects the same parts of the brain that are stimulated by opioids such as heroin.

Chocolate isn't the only food with addictive qualities. A number of other foods, including cheese, have also been found to stimulate opioid receptors. Some foods—mainly sugar and refined carbohydrates—cause alternating surges and drops in glucose (blood sugar) that stimulate appetite and food cravings.

This is why it's not enough to deal only with calories when you're trying to lose weight—or to feel guilty when you slip off your weight-loss plan. You're probably dealing with addictions, which means you have to work hard to break the cravings cycle. Here's some help.

Sugar addiction   Some recent diets emphasize "carbohydrate addiction." This is a little misleading. You know anyone who's addicted to, say, broccoli? The carbs that people really crave are crackers, pastries, and fries. Yes, these foods are carbohydrates, but the true addiction is to the concentrated sugars in them. When you eat highly processed, high-glycemic carbohydrates, glucose floods the bloodstream. The pancreas churns out insulin to get rid of the excess sugar. The insulin then removes so much of it that you experience a glucose plunge. That's about the time you start craving still more sugar.

To stop this cycle:

- Eat low-glycemic, high-fiber carbohydrates such as beans, whole grains, vegetables, and so on. One study found that doing nothing more than eating regular, slow-digesting oatmeal instead of the instant kind caused participants to snack about 35 percent less throughout the day.

- Eat more protein. This controls your hunger and improves the ability of insulin to remove sugar from the blood, causing less precipitous spikes and falls.

- Eat enough and eat often. As long as you're eating healthy foods, frequent meals stabilize blood sugar (and insulin) and reduce out-of-control cravings.

"Death by Chocolate"   For millions of Americans, chocolate is among the leading sources of extra (and excess) calories. Hard to give it up? You bet! Apart from its opioid-like effects, chocolate contains addictive caffeine, a stimulating substance called *theobromine*, and a drug-like chemical called *phenylethylamine*. It also has chemical compounds that resemble those found in marijuana. No wonder so many people call themselves chocolate addicts or chocoholics.

■ The average chocolate bar has about 200 calories and more than 10 grams of fat. That's a lot of extra calories, especially if you eat one or more every day. *Helpful hint*: Buy individually wrapped chocolates, such as Hershey's Dark Chocolates, for easier portion control. You can still occasionally indulge your chocolate tooth while keeping the calorie count down and helping your heart at the same time.

■ Monthly estrogen swings are often behind chocolate cravings. If you eat more fiber-rich foods and cut back on fat around the time of your period, you'll smooth out hormonal fluctuations that trigger these cravings.

■ Maintain or increase your regular exercise schedule in the cold months to combat feeling low. Winter depression often stimulates the urge for chocolate and other sweets.

Cheese   Like chocolate and sugar, cheese triggers a class of opiates (*casomorphins*) that can be highly addictive. When you consider that a thumb-sized piece of cheese packs about 15 grams of fat and 200 calories, you can see why cheese binges can really put on the pounds.

■ You don't have to give up cheese to curtail cravings or calories, but you do have to eat less. Try dairy-free soy cheese as a substitute. It provides real cheese texture and flavor without the addictive properties.

- Order your burgers without cheese at the fast-food counter. When getting a pizza, ask that it be made with half the usual amount of cheese.

- When you have to have cheese, look for reduced-fat products such as low-fat mozzarella and ricotta. Better yet, substitute other foods that give the same creamy mouth feel without all the fat and calories, such as avocado or yogurt.

Doesn't all this sound easy? I told you it would be. And there are plenty of other success tips like this in the pages ahead. I promise: You don't need to go on a diet to lose weight and improve your health—and you won't have to give up the foods you love.

CHAPTER 4

The Fast-Food Diet Restaurant-by-Restaurant Guide

L et me throw a few surprising food statistics at you. One-third of the total calories in the American diet come from restaurant food. About 10 percent of that is made up by fast food.

Nearly 20 percent of Americans are hard-core "fast foodies," meaning they eat convenience or fast food *every day*.

Despite the admittedly weak efforts of the fast-food chains to introduce healthier foods, the three most popular menu items haven't budged over the decades: french fries, soft drinks, and, of course, the almighty hamburger.

When you consider that you can easily blow most of a day's fat and calorie allotment in a fifteen-minute lunch—a Quarter Pounder with double cheese at McDonald's can overload your system with 730 calories and 40 grams of fat—it's hard to imagine that anyone could eat fast food with any regularity and still lose weight. But I've already promised you that it is true. This chapter will show you how. Anyone who follows the simple, easy tips in this book can succeed. In chapter 7, I give you a Six-Week Fast-Food Diet eating plan that's a no-brainer. All of the calories, fat, and carbohydrates have already been figured out for you. Just follow along every day and you'll lose weight without feeling deprived.

Waiting for the chains to change could take a very long time. This isn't to say they haven't given it a try. Burger King, for example, came out with the Veggie Burger, and McDonald's introduced the Go Active! Happy Meal (which has since been dropped). But the fast-food industry is in the business of giving people what they want. And what people want (for the moment, anyway) are the familiar flavors, textures, and menu items they've come to know, love, and crave. While surveys do show that North Americans are taking steps to improve their diets, they are mainly cleaning up their acts at home. When they eat out, they want a treat. This book lets you have your cake and eat it, too—one that makes it possible to lose weight on the fast foods you crave. This book is also a handy reference source for the nutritional facts about your favorite fast-food snacks. These data—calorie content, grams of fat, percentage of refined carbs, and other important facts—aren't printed on the cups and wrappers and french fry boxes. And good luck trying to find a nutritional chart on the wall of Burger King, Kentucky Fried Chicken, or most other fast-food restaurants.

Even when the fast-food chains promote menu items as being particularly nutritious, they have a tendency to exaggerate a bit. For example, you'll often see chicken on their menus. Chicken is a healthful alternative to beef, right? Fast-food marketing departments certainly want you to think so. But the proof is in the preparation. Wendy's Homestyle Chicken Strips Salad topped with ranch dressing, for one, delivers

670 calories and 45 grams of fat. Eat that for lunch every day and you'd gain more weight than if you ate their burgers.

My intention is to help you find nutritious, good-tasting, and diet-smart foods at the fast-food counter. And I'm talking not only about salads, although some fast-food salads deserve a second look. Every one of the top chains has broadened its menu to include items with reasonable levels of fat and calories. You can easily fulfill *some* of the requirements of a truly healthful diet—low-glycemic carbs, lots of produce and fiber, more healthy fats, and less of the saturated kind—without ever preparing a meal at home, not that I recommend you do that. But nearly everyone can lose weight and still enjoy their favorite fast-food meals with a little know-how.

If you know how to tinker with your order, you can avoid gaining an additional ounce of weight. Even better, you can achieve the kinds of fat-and-calorie savings that can quickly knock back your daily total by *at least* 10 percent. That might not sound like much, but a mere 10 percent reduction in daily calories for the average person adds up to about 200 calories. You'll never even notice that. Suppose you eat five take-out meals a week. That's 1,000 calories saved—the equivalent of nearly a third of a pound a week, or more than a pound a month. Instead of having gained weight at the end of the year, you will have lost 12 pounds.

I realize that losing 12 pounds in a year doesn't sound like much, but look at what you had to do to achieve these results. *Almost nothing!* If you follow more of the easy tips in this book, you'll lose more—a lot more. I've designed this eating plan so you can lose 100 pounds in a year's time if you need to, without giving up fast food or joining a gym. And if you're really motivated, you can lose even more.

Suppose you're driving home from work. There's a McDonald's, a Wendy's, and a Burger King on one side of the street.

On the other side there's KFC, Taco Bell, Subway, and Arby's. In the middle—well, you know what I mean! There are a lot of take-out joints out there. Which will you choose—and what will you order when you get there? Here's some help.

Arby's

No matter how you slice it, roast beef is lower in total and saturated fat than its grease-fried burger cousins. But that doesn't go for the special sauces and gooey toppings. Order your roast beef sandwiches plain and you can easily save 100 or more calories. On average, the Arby's menu offers some of the lowest-calorie meals in the fast-food world. The fat content, however, is similar to others unless you hold the toppings. Here are six good choices from Arby's.

Regular Roast Beef   It's not the biggest sandwich in town, and it might not be enough food if you have a bigger-than-average appetite. But for most folks, one is all it takes—and it's lean enough to have every day. (If you order the Jr. Roast Beef instead, you'll knock off 50 calories.) Vital stats: *320 calories, 13 grams total fat, 6 grams saturated fat.*

Chicken Breast Filet   It's quite a bit higher in calories and total fat than the Regular Roast Beef, but it's lower in saturated fat—good news if you're trying to lower cholesterol and keep your heart in the safety zone. This sandwich comes with leaf lettuce and tomatoes, pushing your fresh veggie intake a little higher. Given the relatively high calories, you'll want to eat a little leaner throughout the day. Vital stats: *500 calories, 25 grams total fat, 4 grams saturated fat.*

Market Fresh Roast Turkey and Swiss   The reason I like this sandwich is that it's a truly rich meal—almost sinfully so—yet it doesn't clock off the chart in the fat-and-calorie department. Don't get me wrong: You wouldn't want one every day. But for a treat that won't totally bust your diet? Go for it! Vital stats: *720 calories, 27 grams total fat, 7 grams saturated fat.*

Market Fresh Chicken Salad   This is one of those dishes in life that has to be creamy—which means, of course, more fat than you'd want to consume very often. But it has a good variety of those nutritious ingredients (grapes, apples, and pecans, for example) that you need to shed pounds and stay healthy. Vital stats: *770 calories, 38 grams total fat, 9 grams saturated fat.*

Santa Fe Salad   This isn't the healthiest salad on the Arby's menu, but it's the one most people are likely to order—and still feel like they got a "real" meal. You can skim quite a few calories if you hold the cheese and go easy on the dressing. Vital stats: *520 calories, 29 grams total fat, 9 grams saturated fat.*

Sourdough Egg 'n Cheese   Whether you're trying to start the day right, or you just have a taste for a piece of wholesome bread topped with something nice, this breakfast sandwich is among the leaner fast-food choices. Vital stats: *330 calories, 16 grams total fat, 6 grams saturated fat.*

Burger King

It's the country's second-largest burger chain, and the first to dish up a vegetarian burger—with reduced-fat mayo, no less. But hold the applause. Even though the Veggie Burger is a winner, with only 429 calories, the thrust of Burger King's menu is decidedly toward *bigger*, *more*, and *higher*. The Double Whopper with Cheese hovers around 1,000 calories, with a knock-down 27 grams of saturated fat. The Old Fashioned

Vanilla Milkshake is almost a meal by itself, with 700 calories and 41 grams of fat (26 of them the artery-clogging saturated kind).

To be fair, Burger King's fat-and-calorie bombs aren't any worse than the competitions'. They just seem to have more of them. There isn't a lot on the BK menu that fits comfortably into any reasonable diet, but you can cherry-pick and find a few things that are more or less reasonable. Load up your sandwiches with onions, tomatoes, and lettuce, and you'll push your vegetable and fiber intake in a healthier direction without adding substantially to the calories. Here are six good choices from BK.

BK Veggie Burger   This is by far the leanest item on the menu—and in fact one of the healthiest choices at any of the fast-food chains. It tastes pretty good, too. Vital stats: *420 calories, 16 grams total fat, 3 grams saturated fat*. Get it without mayo, and you can shave 80 calories off the total.

Original Whopper Jr.   When you have a hankering for a burger and a small size doesn't cut it, consider this down-sized version of the original Whopper. It isn't too bad—but you'll still want to eat leaner foods at home to compensate for the relatively high fat total. Vital stats: *390 calories, 27 grams total fat, 7 grams saturated fat*.

Chicken Whopper Sandwich   It's leaner than the beef Whopper, especially if you get it without mayo. And it's filling enough for just about any appetite. Vital stats: *570 calories, 25 grams total fat, 4.5 grams saturated fat*.

Fire-Grilled Chicken or Shrimp Garden Salad   This is proof that a salad doesn't have to leave you hungry. This flavorful meat-and-garden salad is filling enough for a full meal, and healthy enough to enjoy without worrying about calories. If you get it with shrimp, you'll also give yourself a blast of those healthy omega-3 fatty acids. Vital stats: *310 calories, 18 grams total fat, 4 grams saturated fat.*

Chili   It's a small bowl (7.5 ounces), so it's not going to fill you up. But it makes a great appetizer—and delivers some of those beans that are among the best foods for controlling appetite and losing weight. Vital stats: *190 calories, 8 grams total fat, 3 grams saturated fat.*

Angus Steak Burger   I can already hear what you're asking: "What the heck is a steak burger doing in a 'healthy' diet?" Well, I've included it for two reasons: (1) It's sometimes mighty tempting to really satisfy your craving for meat. (2) While this isn't the leanest choice I've seen, it's better than a lot of the other fast foods out there. Vital stats: *570 calories, 22 grams total fat, 8 grams saturated fat.*

Carl's Jr.

It isn't the biggest fast-food chain, but people who eat at Carl's Jr. say it has some of the best-tasting fast food available. With restaurants throughout the United States and Canada, it's clearly a major player in the fast-food market.

Nutritionally, Carl's Jr. is more or less the same as most take-out restaurants. Much of the menu consists of meals that, in terms of fat, sodium, and calories, will just about blow the lid off your diet (and health). That said, Carl's Jr. has made a decent effort to include foods that will fit pretty well into any weight-loss plan. Here are the five best choices from Carl's Jr.

Charbroiled BBQ Chicken Sandwich   If you haven't eaten all day and your stomach is growling, definitely consider this sandwich. It's a meal in itself—with very reasonable amounts of fat and calories. Vital stats: *370 calories, 4 grams total fat, 1 gram saturated fat.*

Charbroiled Chicken Club Sandwich   When you see the word "club," you know you're dealing with more than a few fat calories. That's okay. There are times when all of us really want something a little on the rich side. As an occasional treat, it could be a lot worse. Vital stats: *550 calories, 23 grams total fat, 7 grams saturated fat.*

Charbroiled Chicken Salad-to-Go   I'm a big fan of lunch and supper salads. The meat provides sufficient amounts of stay-full protein, so you don't get hungry an hour later. And since most of us don't get enough produce in our diets, a salad always deserves top billing. Vital stats: *330 calories, 7 grams total fat, 4 grams saturated fat.*

Broccoli and Cheese   I hesitate to include a side dish that has cheese as a main ingredient. But getting extra broccoli in your diet is always a good thing, so this seems like a reasonable compromise. For a side dish, though, the calories are definitely on the high side. Only get it when you're in the mood for a light meal. If you combine it with a burger or shake, the calorie load starts to get serious. Vital stats: *510 calories, 21 grams total fat, 5 grams saturated fat.*

Carl's Catch Fish Sandwich   Don't confuse this fish dish with the delicately sautéed flounder you might make at home—it's not particularly lean or low in calories. But it does provide omega-3 fatty acids, which we could all use more of. Vital stats: *560 calories, 27 grams total fat, 7 grams saturated fat.*

Kentucky Fried Chicken

Just about every weight-loss expert advises substituting chicken for beef. Chicken has less total fat—and much less saturated fat—than regular ground beef. But when you wrap any chicken in breading and submerge it in a deep-fat fryer, it becomes a Frankenbird. Not long ago, the Federal Trade Commission took KFC to task for claiming in advertisements that two Original Recipe chicken breasts had less fat than a Whopper and were therefore healthier. Turns out they were telling us a "whopper." What the ads didn't mention is that the chicken breasts have three times the trans fat and cholesterol and more than twice the sodium. Oops.

You can peel the skin off fried chicken and knock down the fat by about half—but who's likely to do that? Fortunately, there are a few other things—but only a few—on the menu that can keep calories in a reasonable range. Here are your best choices at KFC.

Oven Roasted Twister   Roasting a bird delivers less fat than frying it. This tender chicken filet, topped with pepper mayo and tomato and wrapped in a tortilla, isn't a perfect pick because the total fat is definitely on the high side. The saturated fat, however, tops out at 4 grams, which isn't too bad. Vital stats: *520 calories, 23 grams total fat, 4 grams saturated fat.*

Baked Beans   The easiest way to get a low-calorie, low-fat meal at KFC is to order from the side menu. By combining beans and corn, you get both a vegetable and legume serving at a single meal. That's as close to perfect as you can get. Vital stats: *230 calories, 1 gram total fat, 1 gram saturated fat.*

Corn on the Cob   I spent quite a bit of time inspecting the menu at KFC to find foods that I could honestly recommend for weight control. There weren't a lot of choices, but corn on the cob certainly fits the bill. Vital stats: *70 calories, 1.5 grams total fat, 0.5 grams saturated fat.*

Mashed Potatoes and Gravy   It's not exactly a meal by itself, but it's one of the reasons people love KFC. This dish is filling and has only one-third as much fat as the potato wedges, and about 110 fewer calories. But not all is bleak on the tater front. While potatoes are guilty of raising insulin (about as much as refined sugar) and adding gravy does boost your fat intake, spuds are rich in the much-needed mineral potassium. So having small portions once or twice a week is far better than ordering fries. Vital stats: *130 calories, 4.5 grams total fat, 1 gram saturated fat.*

McDonald's

It's tougher to find items on the main menu at McDonald's that promote real weight loss and general health. The Big Mac alone, which isn't all that big compared to some of the other burger behemoths out there, delivers 560 calories. To its credit, McDonald's has included quite a few non-burger meals on the menu. Unfortunately, these aren't the things most people want to order. In the meantime, there are a *few* items that won't blow your fat or calorie budget. Here are your best picks at Mickey D's.

Premium Grilled Chicken Classic Sandwich   It's not a total calorie lightweight, but at least the chicken is grilled instead of battered and fried—and if you top it with Newman's Own Low-Fat Family Recipe Italian Dressing, it can easily fit into any weight-loss plan. Vital stats: *470 calories, 9 grams total fat, 2 grams saturated fat.*

Caesar Salad with Grilled Chicken   As with most chicken salads at any of the chains, this one's high in sodium (880 milligrams). So if high blood pressure is something you're dealing with, don't bother. But if your overall sodium intake is good, go for it. This salad is filling, flavorful, and very good for losing weight. Vital stats: *220 calories, 6 grams total fat, 3 grams saturated fat.*

Fruit 'n Yogurt Parfait   With this one, McDonald's has earned a pat on the back. It's a rich-tasting dessert that doesn't act rich. Vital stats: *160 calories, 2 grams total fat, 1 gram saturated fat.*

Sonic

While most fast-food chains have transformed themselves over the decades into sit-down restaurants, Sonic has stayed true to its drive-in roots. It's the nation's largest drive-in chain, with more than three thousand restaurants coast to coast.

You can easily order a meal at Sonic that packs in enough fat and calories to really sink your diet. (You don't even have to walk to pick it up, since carhops deliver orders right to your window.) As with the other fast-food outlets, however, Sonic has made an effort to include some healthier choices. Here are your best menu picks at Sonic.

Chicken Strip Snack   I know, it's not exactly a meal, but if you order it with an iced tea, you'll get enough calories that you won't be starving an hour later. Vital stats: *272 calories, 13 grams total fat, 2 grams saturated fat.*

Jr. Burger   When I eat out, I often look at the children's side of the menu first. These reduced-portion meals are in line with the amount of food that most adults actually need. Besides, why jam in so many calories that you can hardly stay awake afterward? The Jr. Burger is plenty big enough to satisfy any reasonable appetite. Vital stats: *353 calories, 21 grams total fat, 6 grams saturated fat.*

Grilled Chicken Salad   You can't go wrong with this one. But if you drench it with regular ranch dressing, you'll add 28 grams of fat—60 percent more than you'd get in the salad itself! Order this with the Light Original Ranch Dressing, and you'll have a meal you can live with. Vital stats (with light dressing): *475 calories, 24 grams total fat, 8 grams saturated fat.*

Grilled Chicken Wrap   This is one of the few menu items that I'd feel comfortable eating—if not every day, at least once or twice a week. Vital stats: *539 calories, 27 grams total fat, 5 grams saturated fat.*

Regular Chili & Cheese Fries   You wouldn't expect a food that includes the words "cheese" and "fries" to be particularly good for you. This is no exception, but the fat content puts it in the "reasonable" category. Vital stats: *299 calories, 19 grams total fat, 6 grams saturated fat.*

Subway

Earlier I mentioned Subway's slimmed-down spokesman, Jared Fogel, who lost 245 pounds by eating Subway sandwiches and exercising. While I don't recommend a diet as restrictive and, let's be honest, as *boring* as Fogel's, my hat's off to him. He's living proof it can be done. Of all the fast-food chains, Subway offers the best menu for low-fat, low-calorie choices. Those sandwiches, if heaped with mounds of fresh vegetables and served on a whole-grain roll, represent a truly healthful diet. Here are nine excellent choices from Subway.

Turkey Breast Submarine Sandwich (6-inch)   Turkey is always a good choice because it's one of the leaner meats— and if you get it with the whole-wheat bun, you'll have plenty of not-so-high-glycemic carbohydrates to keep your stomach satisfied. Double up on the olives, onions, tomatoes, and other fixings, and you can get a couple of vegetable servings right there. Vital stats: *280 calories, 4.5 grams total fat, 1.5 grams saturated fat.*

Sweet Onion Chicken Teriyaki Sandwich (6-inch) This is another winner because chicken, like turkey, is generally a lean meat. I love the onions on this sandwich—not just because I'm an onion lover, but because onions contain some of the most healthful plant chemicals ever discovered—chemicals that protect the cardiovascular system and, along with other vegetables, help prevent heart attacks. Vital stats: *380 calories, 5 grams total fat, 1.5 grams saturated fat.*

Veggie Delite Sandwich (6-inch) The word "veggie" says it all. You could eat this sandwich every day for the rest of your life and keep your weight right where you want it. The variety of vegetables means lots of antioxidants, vitamins and minerals, and low-glycemic carbohydrates—perfect, in other words, for weight control. Vital stats: *230 calories, 3 grams total fat, 1 gram saturated fat.*

Turkey Breast Wrap Just about every restaurant started offering wraps in response to the low-carb craze. I'm not a fan of low-carb diets, but this wrap is a good choice. Vital stats: *190 calories, 6 grams total fat, 1 gram saturated fat.*

Roast Beef Deli Sandwich (6-inch) With a dab of mustard instead of mayo, you'll keep the total calories down where you want them—and it's more than enough food for just about any appetite. Vital stats: *220 calories, 4.5 grams total fat, 2 grams saturated fat.*

Grilled Chicken Breast and Baby Spinach Salad Big enough for a main meal and lean enough to eat daily without gaining an ounce. In fact, if you substituted this salad for a Big Mac or something similar five times a week, you'd save 2,100 calories, the equivalent of more than half a pound. Vital stats: *140 calories, 3 grams total fat, 1 gram saturated fat.*

New England Style Clam Chowder   Get some heart-healthy omega-3s and stick-to-the-ribs carbs at the same time. Vital stats: *110 calories, 3.5 grams total fat, 0.5 grams saturated fat.*

Roasted Chicken Noodle Soup   Nothing you get in a restaurant will be quite like home cooking, but this bowl of soup comes close. Delicious noodles, aromatic broth, tender chicken—mmm! Vital stats: *60 calories, 1.5 grams total fat, 0.5 grams saturated fat.*

Honey Mustard Ham & Egg on Deli Roll   I'm one of those people who don't think eggs are only for breakfast. This egg-on-a-roll sure beats the competition when it comes to weight loss: low in calories and not too much fat. Vital stats: *270 calories, 5 grams total fat, 1.5 grams saturated fat.*

Taco Bell

You probably remember that cute Chihuahua with enormous ears that turned the advertising slogan "Yo quiero Taco Bell" into a cultural catchphrase. The pooch, like the Mexican-style fast-food restaurant itself, seemed to be everywhere. But judging from this corporate canine's sleek profile, he probably wasn't eating much from the hand that fed him.

The core Taco Bell menu, heavy on ground meat and cheese and low on vegetables, won't do your health (or your weight) any good. That said, there are a few menu choices that fall within the good (if not great) zone. Example: Order the tacos "fresco" style—they dress them with salsa instead of cheese and sauce. Here are seven good choices from Taco Bell.

Fresco Style Bean Burrito   It's loaded with low-glycemic beans, which are good for appetite control and have lots of protective antioxidants. It also has 12 grams of fiber, about the American average for an entire day. (The recommended fiber intake is 25 to 35 grams.) Vital stats: *350 calories, 8 grams total fat, 2 grams saturated fat.*

Fresco Style Chicken Ranchero Taco   It's a little on the skimpy side to make a full meal, but it's low enough in calories that you can order two without feeling guilty. Vital stats: *170 calories, 4 grams total fat, 1 gram saturated fat.*

Fresco Style Chalupa Supreme with Chicken   A chalupa, in case you're not familiar with this south-of-the-border standard, is a chewy taco-like shell filled with seasoned ground beef, shredded lettuce, tomatoes, and a variety of cheeses. And you get to eat the bowl! It's not the leanest food you can find, but not too bad, either. Vital stats: *310 calories, 14 grams total fat, 3.5 grams saturated fat.* If you substitute beef for chicken, the calorie count goes up only marginally, but you'll get an extra 4 grams of total fat and an extra 1.5 grams of saturated fat.

Ranchero Chicken Soft Taco   When you're ordering Mexican-style food at any restaurant, it's always a good idea to get soft tacos because they're not dragged through oil. Taco Bell's soft taco—no cheese and heavy on the salsa—is a good choice. Vital stats: *140 calories, 4 grams total fat, 1 gram saturated fat.*

Burrito Supreme-Steak   If you order from the "fresco" side of the menu, you'll get more than enough beef to satisfy your appetite (and taste buds), without consuming gut-busting levels of calories or fat at the same time. Vital stats: *350 calories, 9 grams total fat, 2.5 grams saturated fat.*

Chicken Enchilada   This Mexican classic is a total diet-breaker at most restaurants. Not only are the tortillas dredged in oil, but they're typically loaded with mountains of cheese and sour cream. This enchilada—again, from the "fresco" side of the menu—is a very acceptable alternative. Vital stats: *250 calories, 5 grams total fat, 1.5 grams saturated fat.*

Fresco Style Tostada   This is another traditional fat-bomb that Taco Bell has managed to make a little leaner. Once you strip out the cheese and add the salsa, you get extra bursts of flavor and a serious drop in calories. Vital stats: *200 calories, 6 grams total fat, 1 gram saturated fat.*

Wendy's

The fifth-largest restaurant chain, Wendy's has done a pretty good job of catering to weight-conscious customers. Most of the menu items, as you'd expect from a burger chain, are devoted to the usual high-calorie, fat-drenched standards. The Big Bacon Classic, for example, boasts 580 calories and 29 grams of fat, nearly half of them saturated. Throw in a shake and you can pretty much count on blowing your calorie budget for the day. But Wendy's, unlike many of the other fast-food chains, offers a good selection of healthier options. Here are five good choices from Wendy's.

Ultimate Chicken Grill Sandwich   The word "ultimate" suggests this is a meal in itself—and it is. It's topped with nutritious romaine instead of the usual iceberg lettuce, and it comes on a kaiser roll. It's an excellent choice for calorie control as well as good taste. Vital stats: *360 calories, 7 grams total fat, 1.5 grams saturated fat.*

Mandarin Chicken Salad   When you're in the mood for a light lunch, this is a good option (it comes with a breadstick, which helps round out the meal). It has a good selection of ingredients, though I wish they'd give up on the iceberg lettuce, which is a nutritional lightweight, and use more of the vitamin-filled spring mix. Vital stats: *170 calories, 2 grams total fat, 0.5 grams saturated fat.*

Small Chili (8-ounce)   If you combine it with a salad, you'll get more than enough calories to tide you over until the next meal. The fat content isn't exactly rock-bottom, but it's well within the acceptable range. Vital stats: *220 calories, 6 grams total fat, 2.5 grams saturated fat.*

Sour Cream & Chives Baked Potato   Hold the sour cream and top it off with their chili instead, and you've got a belly-filling meal that's as good as it gets in fast-food land. Add a side salad and feel proud of yourself. You've cracked the code! Vital stats: *320 calories, 4 grams total fat, 2 gram saturated fat.*

Broccoli & Cheese Baked Potato   The cheese on this one drives up the calories a bit, but who can say no to an extra serving of broccoli? As with all of the cabbage-family vegetables, broccoli is jammed with chemical compounds that are among the most potent ever discovered for preventing disease, including cancer. Vital stats: *340 calories, 3.5 grams total fat, 1 gram saturated fat.*

Wienerschnitzel

You can now buy low-fat hot dogs in supermarkets, and it's possible to get a reasonably lean dog in a take-out joint. Not easy, but possible.

I can't bring myself to totally condemn hot dogs. Just about everyone loves them, and they're less likely than their burger cousins to come slathered in mayo or other creamy, calorie-drenched dressings. Low-calorie? Nope. Low-fat? Nope. Good for you? Nope. But hey, life is short. What else are you going to eat on the Fourth of July! Here are their three best menu items.

Turkey Chili Dog　Go ahead, load on the toppings: onions, relish, sauerkraut. A dog with the works is a great way to get some of your daily vegetables—and by holding the cheese, you'll keep the fat and calorie load in the safety zone. Vital stats: *270 calories, 11 grams total fat, 3 grams saturated fat.*

Mustard Dog on a Pretzel Bun　Okay, it's not exactly low in sodium—but then, few hot dogs are. As long as you aren't dealing with high blood pressure, this isn't a bad choice. Vital stats: *400 calories, 15 grams total fat, 5 grams saturated fat.*

Kraut Dog　Sauerkraut is among the foods we should all eat more of. Cabbage is one of the most chemically active (in a good way) foods there is. Once cabbage is transformed into 'kraut, it's great for your intestinal health. And it counts as a vegetable serving. Vital stats: *260 calories, 12 grams total fat, 4 grams saturated fat.*

Naturally, in a book this size it is impossible to cover every single menu item for all the fast-food restaurants in North America. Besides, many franchises are continually changing menu items, sometimes for the better. In fact, as customers like you begin to make wiser, healthier selections, menus will change quickly. To keep up with these new additions and menu innovations, check in with our free Web site at www .thefastfooddiet.com.

The Top 10 Calorie-Cutting Secrets

1. **Trust the chicken**　There are always exceptions, of course. Fast-food chicken is mostly off the chart in terms

of salt, and can be mighty high in fat and calories if it's fried or breaded. Those caveats aside, most chicken is leaner than beef. A six-inch Oven Roasted Chicken Breast Sandwich at Subway has 330 calories and 5 grams of total fat. The Double Cheeseburger at McDonald's is a smaller sandwich, but has 460 calories and 23 grams of fat. Chicken is usually a safe bet.

2. **Skin the bird**   Most of the fat in fried chicken resides in the skin. The next time you pick up a bucketful of KFC, pull off the skin along with the breading. It will cut the fat load by about half.

3. **Pass (on) the fries**   About 80 percent of customers order fries as a side dish to accompany a burger or chicken sandwich. Yet those fries have about the same number of calories—and often more fat—as the main dish. Worse, a hefty percentage of the fat is of the deadly trans-fat kind. If you can't give up fries entirely, at least eat them rarely— and cut back on fat and calories elsewhere during the day.

4. **Lean toward roast beef**   A roast beef sandwich isn't automatically lean, especially when it's loaded with a creamy dressing. But as a rough and ready rule, the roast beef is generally a leaner sandwich than a hamburger. A Jr. Roast Beef Sandwich at Arby's has 4 grams of fat, while the average burger has about 9 grams.

5. **Easy on the cheese**   You don't lose much flavor when you strip the cheese off a hamburger, but you do lose an impressive amount of fat and calories. Cheese is nearly pure fat. A slice of cheddar, for example, gets 74 percent of its calories from fat. If you've been ordering a burger with cheese a couple times a week, just holding the cheese could save you 30 to 40 calories and 3 to 4 grams of fat each time.

6. **Don't get the "special meals"** Sure, it's economical to get the Value Meal at Burger King or McDonald's, but your waistline and arteries won't like you for it. The combined calories in a burger, fries, and soft drink can easily top 1,000 to 1,200 calories—and the saturated fat can add up to three-quarters or more of the recommended daily limit. The "bargain meals" aren't really a bargain if you care about your health and your weight. You're better off ordering à la carte.

7. **Score with salads** You don't have to make it a daily habit, but choosing a salad is one of the most reliable ways to eat regularly at the chains and still control your weight. Most of the chains offer salads that have gone way beyond lettuce. You can have Caesar, mixed greens, or grilled chicken and know that you're consuming only a fraction of the calories that you'd get from the burger and fries. That's assuming, of course, that you don't drench them in dressing, which can push the calorie-and-fat content back into burger range.

8. **Do without the toppings** It doesn't matter if your idea of a topping is the ranch dressing on salad, the mayo on a burger, or the cream cheese on a bagel. Virtually every topping, with the exception of those labeled low- or reduced-fat, is a fat-and-calorie heavyweight, adding some 50 to 100 calories (or more) to every meal you eat.

9. **Load up on the fixings** There are some toppings you should insist on: a mound of tomatoes, onions, lettuce, green pepper, cucumbers, or anything else that will fit between two slices of bread. You can think of produce as the core of a healthy diet—low in calories, high in fiber, and jammed with high-powered nutrients and antioxidants.

Undress Those Salad Calories

One of the most effective weight-loss strategies is to graze more at salad bars in restaurants and supermarkets. You'll find a remarkable selection of healthy greens, whole-grain salads, cold bean dishes, and just about everything else you need for low-calorie, high-antioxidant meals. But those dressings, if you aren't careful, can derail the best diet and send it careening down the fat tracks. In fact, you can get more fat and calories from a drenching of dressing than you'd get from a Quarter Pounder with fries.

Nearly all dressings, with the exception of those labeled fat-free or low- or reduced-fat, pack some serious calories. Moderation!

Dressing (2 tbsp.)	Fat (grams)	Calories
Blue Cheese	16	149
Dijon	17	150
French	20	185
Italian	14	145
Ranch	16	160
Roquefort	12	120
Thousand Island	18	180

10. **Skip the sodas**   Sugary sodas contain empty calories and set you up for insulin resistance and diabetes and are also the fast track to weight gain.

Battle of the Salads

The ideal diet for the fastest possible weight loss (and good health generally) features as many vegetables and fruits as you

can eat. One of the easiest ways to load up on produce is to eat
a salad with (or for) lunch or dinner. Or both. Unfortunately,
quite a few of the fast-food outlets dish up salads that are
higher in salt than just about anything on the main menu. They
aren't always so great on the fat and calories, either. Take
Burger King's Tender Crisp Salads. Those fried chicken strips
served over greens drive the calorie count to more than 500
and the total fat to 22 grams. Eat a few of those "healthy" salads a week, and you'll gain as much weight as you would if
you stuck to the burgers and shakes.

There are some good (and good-tasting) salads to be found,
and I highly recommend them. Just don't ruin a good thing by
slathering on the high-fat ranch, blue cheese, Thousand Island,
or other creamy dressings. You'll do better to stick with
vinaigrette—or at least use as little of the other dressings as
you can. Here's a look at how the salads compare at the
different chains.

Burger King's Fire-Grilled Caesar Salads   They're made
with nutritious romaine instead of iceberg lettuce, and
include tomatoes, carrots, onion, and cucumber, and come
topped with either grilled chicken or grilled shrimp. At 190
calories and reasonable amounts of fat (7 grams for the
chicken, 10 grams for the shrimp), they're among the
healthiest meals you can find anywhere.

McDonald's Caesar Salad with Grilled Chicken   This is
probably your best weight-loss choice at McDonald's. This
salad contains only 220 calories and 6 grams of fat. Forget
the salad with crispy chicken. The fried meat more than doubles the fat content and kicks in an additional 80 calories.

Subway's Grilled Chicken Breast and Baby Spinach Salad   A
definite winner. Of all the salad greens, spinach is probably

Who's King of the Fries?

Can you guess the most popular vegetable in America? Hands down, it's the french fry. The average American downs almost 30 pounds of them in a year! French fry calories alone explain why North America (especially our kids) has a serious weight problem.

An order of fast-food fries contains massive amounts of saturated fat, as well as trans fats. This double whammy can send your cholesterol soaring and seriously damage your heart and arteries. A large order of fries easily contains upward of 500 calories. Do any of the fast-food chains sell healthy french fries? Nope—but some are worse than others. In descending order of infamy, they are:

Burger King   A king-size order has a whopping 600 calories, 30 grams of total fat, and 16 grams of saturated fat—and 1,140 milligrams of salt. That's w-a-y too much.

Wendy's   The Biggie-size order doesn't deserve the cute name. Munch down a few of these every week and you'll be "living large," as kids like to say—only not in the way they mean. The count: 490 calories, 28 grams of total fat, and 5 grams of saturated fat.

McDonald's   People who love french fries swear by McDonald's. So, presumably, do cardiac surgeons. A large order has 520 calories, 25 grams of total fat, and 5 grams of saturated fat.

KFC   Okay, they're not really fries; they call them "potato wedges." They deserve a mention because they're almost dainty compared to the competition, with 240 calories, 12 grams total fat, and 3 grams of saturated fat.

the best pick for sheer nutritional oomph—and it wilts nicely under the warm chicken. With 300 calories and 3 grams of fat, it's worth putting in your sights.

Wendy's Mandarin Chicken Salad   It's almost as lean as you can get, with only 2 grams of fat and 170 calories. The Mandarin orange slices are a healthy touch. Not quite a full meal, but close.

CHAPTER 5

Smart Sit-Down Dining

There's more to dining out than fast-food restaurants. Chain restaurants such as Applebee's, Olive Garden, and Bennigan's are becoming almost as ubiquitous as the golden arches. Today there are nearly two hundred thousand "tableside" restaurants in the United States, a figure that continues to grow almost weekly. Like fast-food outlets, these dining establishments can be dietary minefields when it comes to managing your weight. They can blow up your best efforts (and your waistline) with menu items and hidden ingredients that contain an explosive number of calories—so many that the bathroom scale will show the results in a hurry.

But things are starting to change. Seven out of ten adults surveyed by the National Restaurant Association believe that there are more nutritious foods available in these restaurants than in the past. Nearly all of these chains have added healthier options to their menus, such as Applebee's Weight Watchers selections, Chili's It's Your Choice Program, and Red Lobster's Lighthouse Menu.

It's definitely a move in the right direction. About 46 percent of North Americans eat out *every day*. At any one of the sit-down chains, you can suck down at least 1,000 calories, along with an entire day's worth of saturated fat and salt, without even touching the side dishes or dessert. How so? One of the biggest problems is the sheer size of the servings. In a "battle of the bargains," the restaurant industry has shifted almost entirely to 12-inch plates. The standard 10-inchers, it seems, don't hold enough food for our new supersize mentality. The calories saved by ordering a "lite" entrée won't begin to make up for those consumed in the new humungous portions.

Our notion of a normal serving is distorted by decades of upsizing. It's almost impossible to accurately gauge if a serving size is small, normal, or extraordinary. Even the pros get confused. About ten years ago, researchers from New York University and the Center for Science in the Public Interest had the clever idea of putting various portion sizes in front of nutritionists to see if they were any better at estimating servings than the rest of us. They showed the nutritionists six meals: lasagna, grilled chicken, Caesar salad, a tuna salad sandwich, a burger with onion rings, and a porterhouse steak dinner. Asked to guess the amount of fat and calories in each dish, the nutritionists' minds boggled! They *underestimated* calorie contents by an average of 37 percent and the fat content by 49 percent. For example, they guessed that the tuna sandwich had 375 calories, when in fact it had 720!

Proper portion sizes are clearly part of the weight-loss equation. Another equally important aspect is what you get in the food you order at these restaurants—and what's missing. Want saturated fat, trans fat, and salt? Pack up the family and head to Chili's, Applebee's, or any of the other chains. A fried seafood platter at Red Lobster, replete with fries, can dump 2,000 or more calories into your breadbasket—plus enough artery-clogging gunk and salt to guarantee Ivy League educations for some cardiologist's children.

The foods that make it easier to lose weight, such as beans, whole grains, and fresh vegetables, are still harder to find.

Fat in a Glass

Many of us enjoy a glass (or two) of wine with meals. Wine, like any other brightly colored food, is replete with heart-friendly antioxidants and other chemical compounds that can help you live longer and healthier.

But there's also a downside. I'm referring not to alcohol abuse, which can be a concern, but to the calories. Alcohol is chemically similar to fat, with about 7 calories per gram. No matter how much you skimp on portions or deny yourself the creamy sauce, having a few glasses of wine, beer, or liquor will drop all of those calories right back in the tank. Here's the lowdown:

- Beer, 12 ounces: about 146 calories
- Vodka, gin, rum, whiskey, or tequila, 2 ounces: about 128 calories
- Red or white wine, 7 ounces: about 85 and 80 calories, respectively
- Cordials: 146 to 186 calories per serving

It's okay to enjoy a glass of wine with dinner or to have a cocktail or an after-dinner brandy. Just make sure you savor every sip to make it last. Responsible drinking isn't only about staying sober, it's also about keeping your weight where you want it. Remember, when it comes to alcohol, less is more.

Usually you have to request them—while also cutting back on the heavily fried and supersized nutritional disasters that we've gotten used to.

Eat Lean, Eat Well

It's not difficult to eat lean and healthfully at almost any restaurant chain—but you must be proactive. This means ordering from the "lighter fare" or "healthy choices" side of the menu—or, if these aren't available, requesting a more diet-conscious preparation of the regular dishes, such as less salt and less added fat, and grilling and steaming rather than frying and sautéing. In the past, many of the so-called healthy meals offered by restaurants *were* pretty bad. I knew when I created this diet that it had to include a wide variety of foods so that boredom never has a chance to set it. Today, it isn't necessary to trade "delicious" for "healthy." You simply need to shift the balance in a healthier direction by eating more of the foods that fill you up with fewer calories and less of the foods that pack on the pounds. Sounds easy—and it is!

Just beware. The restaurant chains, with a few exceptions, don't design their menus with healthy eating in mind. Quite the opposite: they load up most of the expensive dishes with fat, salt, and sugar because that's what consumers are used to—and are willing to pay more for. You'll certainly save money by ordering from the low-cal side of the menu in addition to saving yourself 40 to 50 percent of consumed calories. You'll also get less saturated fat because the restaurants have to trim back on butter or vegetable shortenings to hit those advertised low-calorie limits. And you'll find more vegetables on your plate, which are naturally low in calories. Don't worry about leaving hungry. You won't. Eating lean protein, healthier fats, and low-glycemic carbohydrates, such as beans and vegetables, will fill you up without overloading your system with unnecessary calories. You can even have seconds.

Let's take a look at some of the ways you can gradually (and painlessly) eat well and still lose weight at today's most popular chains. The listings and examples that follow represent only a portion of the healthy possibilities. Check our free Web site, www.thefastfooddiet.com, for regular updates.

Trade the Saturated Fat for Omega-3s and Olive Oil

Whether you're eating out or eating in, olive oil and fish fats (the omega-3s) should comprise the majority of the fats in your foods. And you don't need a lot to reap their benefits. For olive oil, one to two tablespoons a day is plenty. Try to not cook with olive oil because it doesn't hold up well to high heat, which damages some of its protective compounds. You're better off drizzling it over vegetables or grain dishes, or mixing it in salad dressing. When you're dining out, dip a small piece of bread in that little saucer of olive oil rather than help yourself to the butter. Delicious! For omega-3s, one to two fish servings a week just about take care of it. Here are the best choices.

Applebee's   The regular menu is typical of most of the sit-down chains. Just one appetizer (say, the fried mozzarella sticks) can cost you 830 calories and more saturated fat than you want to think about. The Weight Watchers part of the menu, on the other hand, is about as good as you can get. Check out the Grilled Tilapia with Mango Sauce. Tilapia, a farm-raised fish, isn't a great pick for omega-3s because it's a little on the lean side, but it still provides enough to count toward one of your weekly fish servings. With 320 calories, it's a top selection. Their Grilled Shrimp Skewer

Salad is another good choice for omega-3s. It also includes generous amounts of snap peas, onions, and salad greens. Healthy fats plus fresh vegetables—that's a healthful weight-loss combo!

Chili's   Take a look at the items on their Guiltless Grill: plenty of choices, not much saturated fat, and at least one tasty way to bump up your healthy fat intake. Start with the Guiltless Salmon. Salmon has more omega-3s than just about any other fish. And like other fatty fish, it takes on a delicious char and develops a rich smoked flavor when cooked on the grill. A portion only has 480 calories and 3 grams of saturated fat.

T.G.I. Friday's   I'm not a big fan of the Atkins-style diet because it allows way too much saturated fat. On the plus side, it does emphasize low-glycemic carbs along with plenty of healthy fats. T.G.I. Friday's teamed up with Atkins to create a healthier (if not always low-calorie or low-fat) menu. Get your omega-3s from the Key West Tilapia. It comes with fresh roasted vegetables, which you can splash with olive oil for a richer flavor along with the healthy olive-oil antioxidants.

Think Slow Carbs—Not Low Carbs

Between 40 percent and 50 percent of the calories in your diet should come from low-glycemic carbohydrates. I've already explained why they're so critical for weight loss. One quick caveat: The bread that's served at most chain restaurants has been processed to within an inch of its glycemic life. A brown loaf isn't necessarily whole-grain. Ask the waiter before digging to the bottom of the breadbasket. If it's not true whole-grain bread, eat it sparingly.

Red Lobster   Their Lighthouse Menu features foods that are reasonably low in calories. It lists calories, plus fat and fiber content, which makes it easy to see what you're getting. Red Lobster is obviously a good choice for eating one of your weekly fish meals (as long as you avoid battered-and-fried anything). This is mainly a seafood restaurant; the carbohydrate pickings are on the scant side. Two that deserve attention are the Seasoned Broccoli and Wild Rice Pilaf. The pilaf is a good choice because whole grains are high in chromium, which works with insulin to transport glucose into your body's cells.

Olive Garden   Look for the little olive leaves on the menu. These call attention to lower-fat choices. If you start your meal with the minestrone soup, you'll get beans, legumes, and vegetables, which is like hitting the weight-loss tri-fecta! Also, research shows that starting a meal with a soup appetizer reduces the total calories you're likely to consume overall.

Eat Your Veggies

Your mom was right: eating your veggies is good for you. Nothing's better. Vegetables are the closest thing you can find to a long-life guarantee: high in fiber and low in fat and calories. It's almost impossible not to lose weight if you make an effort to load your diet with colorful veggies. From a weight-loss perspective, they're the next-best thing to a miracle pill. They fill you up fast, so you're less likely to load up on other, higher-calorie foods. Just as important, the richly colored hues indicate the presence of thousands of plant-based chemicals and healing compounds called *antioxidants*. These drive down disease rates, while keeping the brain and heart functioning at peak capacity.

More Oil, Less Bread

Many restaurants feature a basket of bread and a little dish of butter. It's a hard combination to resist, but what about the calorie load from this fat-and-carb treat? Remember, bread can push your body's capacity for fat storage too high.

Ask for some olive oil instead. It can actually *reduce* the total calories you consume. University of Illinois researchers gave 341 volunteers equal amounts of bread with either olive oil or butter. The olive-oil dippers really drenched the bread, getting 26 percent more fat per slice than those in the butter group. Yet the butter eaters just couldn't quit. They ate more bread and wound up consuming 17 percent more total calories.

Let me tell you a secret. You can dine out three or four days a week and never gain an ounce. You can even eat out every day and still maintain a healthy weight. The key is to load up on fresh vegetables and fruits. Order them with every meal, and definitely keep your refrigerator well stocked so you can cook with them. Most people who do this at home easily keep their weight under control.

Remember, I'm not telling you any of this to get you to overhaul the way you normally eat. Very few of us, when we treat ourselves to a good meal, think mainly of the health benefits of what's on the end of the fork. We go out to enjoy and to celebrate life. That's fine. As long as you heed the 80/20 Rule, you'll have plenty of room for indulgences. And by making some small, simple changes—such as simply adding extra tomatoes to a chicken sandwich—you'll find that your weight will naturally drift closer to where you want it and the long-term health benefits will accrue like compound interest at the bank.

Go Easy on the Dairy

One thing that this diet doesn't emphasize is large amounts of dairy. Contrary to what you usually hear from the dairy industry, none of us really "needs" milk, cheese, or other dairy foods. You'll get plenty of calcium when you bump up your consumption of fresh vegetables. A single serving of kale, for example, provides as much calcium as a glass of milk. There's also some medical evidence that the fat and protein in dairy products actually *promote* osteoporosis by creating an acidic pH environment in the body that must be buffered by pulling calcium out of the bones. It's interesting that in countries where dairy consumption is the highest, so are the rates of osteoporosis. Countries with the lowest dairy consumption have the least osteoporosis.

As for cheese, you're taking a chance with anything that isn't explicitly labeled low-fat. A wedge of cheese might seem like a healthier option than a big slice of chocolate mousse cake, but it's almost pure fat and could easily pack 500 calories!

Whole Grains and Legumes

These are among the most nutritious weight-loss foods you can eat. You can't go wrong by boosting the percentage of your daily calories (and protein) from grains and legumes—these include beans, lentils, soybeans, and peas. They are ideal for weight loss because, besides filling you up on a minimum of calories, their complex sugars convert to glucose in the blood slowly. That means fewer insulin spikes, less conversion to fat, and longer periods without feeling hungry.

A few years ago, it would have been just about impossible to find whole grains or legumes at chain restaurants. Sure, you could ask for whole-wheat toast, but that was about it. These days, you won't have to look very hard. At Panera Bread, for example, you can fill up with a rich-tasting bean soup. Au Bon Pain offers a variety of freshly baked whole-grain breads. And many chains, even those that don't bill themselves as Mexican, offer plenty of bean dishes, such as bean-filled burritos. Of course, not all restaurant vegetables are created equal. By the time they're doused in butter or drenched in some fatty sauce, such as hollandaise or béarnaise, they can load you up with as many calories as the main dish. So if you're already getting a high-fat entrée, try to keep your vegetables lean, steamed, and uncreamed. Here are a few suggestions when you're eating out.

Ruby Tuesday   If I were to open my own restaurant, it would include quite a few of the vegetable sides that are featured on Ruby Tuesday's Smart Eating menu. There are more vegetable choices than you usually find in this kind of place: sautéed zucchini, sugar snap peas, broccoli, and cole slaw. That's a lot of antioxidants and fiber! Unfortunately, some of these dishes are higher in fat than they should be. The broccoli delivers 8 grams, and the creamed spinach packs in 17 grams. Go for the leaner greens. Also on the Smart Eating Menu is a brown rice pilaf that will fill you up. It has only 223 calories. Great choice!

P.F. Chang's   It's one of the few big chains that provide a standard vegetarian menu plus side dishes and entrees (meat and meatless) that are replete with vegetables and whole grains. Try Buddha's Feast Steamed for a main dish. It includes asparagus, black mushrooms, snap peas, baby corn, and other vegetables—all with 1.5 total grams of fat, no saturated fat, and 200 calories. For a side, the steamed vegetable dumplings are a good choice. They're high in calories for an appetizer (300), but contain almost no saturated fat.

Outback   A popular steak house known for its generous servings of super-saturated-fat entrees (along with the famous Bloomin' Onion), it also has a Healthy Weight Loss Menu. You can find vegetable dishes on both the entrée menu (such as the Shrimp and Veggie Platter) and the appetizer side. They also serve steamed vegetables without butter.

Chili's   Most bean and grain dishes at the nation's chains are found on the appetizer or salad side of the menu. At Chili's you can get an honest-to-goodness Black Bean Burger. That's right, a no-meat patty made with black beans and topped with low-fat ranch dressing. It's not super-light at 650 calories, but it has only two grams of saturated fat. And it counts toward one of your daily legume servings as well as a serving of whole grain if you order it on the whole-wheat bun.

Olive Garden   The Pasta e Fagioli is nearly the perfect way to get the good-for-you carbs in vegetables and beans. This Italian classic includes white and red beans, pasta, tomatoes, and a little ground beef. It's a bit high in fat, though, so consider it a now-and-then appetizer or a light entrée.

A Little Know-How Goes a Long Way

When you go out to eat and you order more low-glycemic carbs, ask for more fruits and vegetables, and replace those heart-stopping saturated fats with the healthful fats I've been discussing, you'll lose weight easily because your total calorie intake will drop, while your body's natural fat-burning mechanisms will kick into high gear. This diet is a comfortable fit with the way we really eat (not just the way we should). The truth is, you can't live entirely on restaurant food and have a perfect diet—but you *can* have a very good diet and drop those stubborn pounds along the way.

The American Dietetic Association, the world's largest group of nutritionists, says that there are no good or bad foods but that you should consume a balanced diet with everything in moderation. I tend to agree, though there are certain exceptions, such as trans fat and high fructose corn syrup. Their point, a fair one, is that moderation and balance, choosing a variety of foods from different groups and not overstuffing yourself, are what determine a healthy diet. If your usual diet is healthy, who cares if you dive into a 2,000-calorie steak dinner now and then? But if your diet needs some work, general principles count more than rules. Individual foods or food groups, such as carbs, fats, or sugar, are rarely the whole problem—or the whole answer.

A point often missed is that most of us dine at restaurants quite frequently these days. This is especially true of business-people who travel and entertain often. And in doing so, we find it not always easy to maintain the proper moderation and balance in our diets. Usually, when we eat out, we want it to be a delicious experience. The real challenge is how to satisfy our current food preferences and still lose weight and stay healthy. Following the simple guidelines in this book makes this very doable. My hope is that you will incorporate many of them in your daily life so that your health and weight will take a noticeable turn for the better. Here are a few more table-side tips that can help.

Order what you *don't* eat at home   Eating out is a good chance to round out your diet by ordering things you're unlikely to prepare at home. A lot of us, for example, could do without the smell of fish in the kitchen. It's a great excuse to order fish when you go out. Are grain and bean dishes a little too time-consuming? Let the restaurant do the

Catch of the Day: Just How Healthy Is Fresh Fish?

Millions of Americans are following their doctors' advice to eat more fish. But you've got to be careful. A new study in California's Bay Area found that all the fish tested had mercury levels in excess of the safe limit of 5 parts per billion—and 70 percent had *twice* that level.

Mercury accumulates mainly in large fish at the top of the food chain, such as swordfish, tilefish, shark, and halibut. The evidence isn't conclusive, but some doctors believe that even low levels of mercury may offset the heart-healthy benefits of the omega-3 fatty acids in fish. Is it possible to get the benefits of omega-3s without worrying about mercury? Yes, but it takes some planning. Pick fish that don't accumulate mercury, such as wild salmon, sardines, sole, and cod. Avoid or eat less high-mercury fish, such as swordfish, sea bass, shark, tilefish, halibut, orange roughy, and ahi tuna.

It's also a good idea to ask your waiter if tuna salads are made with chunk light tuna or albacore. Chunk light tuna has two-thirds less mercury. Finally, there's no need to overload your diet from the fish side of the menu. About two weekly servings are enough to get the benefits of omega-3s. A 2-ounce serving of salmon delivers 1 gram of omega-3s, the minimum amount per serving recommended by the American Heart Association for cardiovascular health.

work. You don't make or keep desserts at home? Order the delicious sorbet or the panna cotta. Live a little—and fill in the nutritious gaps in your diet at the same time.

Watch your calorie budget On average, men should eat no more than 1,800 calories a day to lose weight. For women, the ideal is about 1,500. If you're planning a blow-out dinner, be a little careful during the day. Don't starve yourself, because you could end up eating everything but the tablecloth later. Try to cut back a bit at breakfast and lunch so that the big dinner calories don't push you beyond your weight-loss limit.

Start with soup   Don't worry about the extra calories in soup (unless it's cheese- or cream-based). Eating soup is a sure way to lose weight. Studies show that people who eat soup before an entrée tend to be less hungry throughout the day, take in fewer calories at meals, and weigh less than folks who don't eat soup. In fact, people who start a meal with soup tend to take in some 400 fewer daily calories overall.

Choose the leaner meats   I'm not talking about tough-as-a-saddle flank steak. The cuts of meat served in restaurants are uniformly rich and fatty, but some are better than others. For example, a sirloin steak has far fewer calories than a porterhouse.

Visualize portions   A recent survey by the American Institute for Cancer Research found that 26 percent of all adults eat everything that's put in front of them in a restaurant—and restaurants, as we all know, put a lot of food on our plates. Before you order, take a mental picture of what you consider a reasonable serving. Then when your order arrives, separate the portion you're going to eat and save the rest for a take-home box.

Beware of the freebies   No kidding. Those little things that wind up on the table without anyone ordering them—the bread, breadsticks, *amuse bouche*, olives marinated in oil, the dips and little pats of butter—can sneak in a lot more calories than you might think. Nibble the bread as a special treat, dipped in olive oil. Then fold your hands and wait for the main event.

Double-beware of the dressings   The average restaurant salad comes with about four tablespoons of dressing. That may not sound like much, but dressings often provide 50 percent to 80 percent of the calories in tossed salads—and can add about 300 calories. Or consider the sour cream in a baked potato. If they really slather it on (in addition to the butter load) you're looking at *at least* 300 calories—and probably more. Personally, I always prefer my salad with dressing. Ditto for sour cream on a baked potato. You don't have to give them up; just control the calories. Get the salad dressings and other toppings on the side. Dip your fork in the dressing to get the flavor, take a bite, and then dip again. At the end of the meal, you'll have taken in far fewer calories.

Get smarter starters   Those stuffed mushroom caps and clams casino sure taste good. But oh, the fat! Why blow your entire day's calorie budget before you even get to the entrée? Take a little time to browse the appetizers. Start with things like smoked salmon, vegetable soup, a shrimp cocktail, or tomatoes with mozzarella and vinaigrette. They're a lot leaner, not to mention more elegant, than the fried stuff.

Double up on side dishes   They can be among the healthiest foods on the menu and the portions are smaller. Most chains offer items such as steamed vegetables, rice pilaf, and bean soup. If you like the side orders, make a meal of them. Get two or three and skip the higher-calorie entrée entirely.

Make room for marinara   Restaurants like Olive Garden and Macaroni Grill specialize in pastas, which can be a superb way to limit calories and also get an extra serving of grain. It's the pasta sauces you have to watch out for. A tomato-based marinara is a lot lower in fat and calories than a cream or Alfredo sauce. If whole-grain pasta or a mix of white and whole-wheat is available, go for it.

Can the sodas   If you enjoy a soft drink with your dinner—or, like a lot of people, two or three since refills are usually free—you're swigging a lot of unnecessary calories. A 12-ounce soft drink typically has more than nine teaspoons of sugar, and restaurant servings are usually a lot bigger than that. Here's a scary statistic: If you drank a 20-ounce soft drink every day for a year, *you'd gain about 24 pounds from the extra calories!*

Eat lighter at lunch   A lot of folks have one or more business lunches a week, often at chains because it's easy to get in and out in an hour. Those lunches can rack up unwanted calories, especially when you realize that you hardly taste anything because so much talking is going on. These are perfect occasions to order the soup and salad. You won't be so tired when you get back to work and you'll have "saved up" some calories that you can use for a meal you'll really enjoy.

Ordering Well, Eating Well

Finally, many restaurants are beginning to get it. Today they routinely ladle out olive oil, put fresh fruits on dessert menus, and offer quite a few vegetable, grain, and bean dishes. Tofu, veggies, and brown rice on the menu? No one gives them a second look, even if they're not quite ready to give them a try.

Eating with these concepts in mind is more flexible and less restrictive than many of today's trendy diets. Even so, many of my patients look a little confused when I explain this to them. Somehow they've gotten the idea that there are only two kinds of diets: a *perfect* diet, in which you only eat the recommended foods and give up all the "good stuff" in life, and a *failed* diet.

In an ideal world, we'd all load up on health-promoting foods, and skip the rest. But that's not real life. Did you stick to a salad and vegetable plate when you celebrated your anniversary? I wouldn't ask anyone to do that—unless they truly enjoyed it.

I don't know about you, but life without an occasional feast isn't fun to me. No one eats a perfect diet all the time, not even me, and remember, I'm a certified nutritionist. If you have a hankering for a fatty, greasy burger—have it! Doctor's orders. Life is too short to deny yourself a few simple pleasures. It's all about 80/20. As long as you're eating well *most* of the time, there's plenty of room for the occasional blowout.

Increase Your Restaurant Savvy

Eating healthfully in sit-down restaurants isn't tricky at all. Fast-food outlets require a little more careful navigation to avoid getting whacked by the elephantine portions of sugar, salt, and saturated fats. Here are a few more helpful tips when you're dining at a sit-down restaurant.

Grill the waiter   Restaurant chains have gotten pretty good at training the staff to answer questions about what goes into the various dishes. Don't assume that the grilled fish will be completely healthful. Ask first: Does it come dripping in butter? Will the chef prepare it without salt and with a minimum of oil? Can the gravy and dressing be served on the side? Does any of the food contain MSG? (Hint: The "sodium" in monosodium glutamate won't do your blood pressure any good and could give you an MSG headache.) Today's chefs are usually flexible about what they include in or omit from their recipes. But they routinely ladle butter over already cooked fish or vegetables to boost flavors. If you don't want that, tell the waiter. (See "Eleven Questions to Ask the Waiter" on page 89.)

Fish around for good fats   You almost can't go wrong ordering fish, as long as it doesn't come swimming in butter, or caked in a deep-fried mound of breading. The essential fatty acids in fish are good for you, so load up on the seafood side of the menu whenever you can. Even if your dinner companions are in the mood for thick steaks, most steak houses offer a few fish choices.

Request substitutions   Just because the menu says that a dish comes with fries or other sides, don't feel that you're stuck with them. Most restaurants are happy to substitute a salad, an extra serving of broccoli, or a baked potato for those fries. In fact, you can often get a double serving of beans, vegetables, or grains without paying extra. A good rule of thumb when following my weight-loss plan is that roughly half your plate should be reserved for vegetable foods of one kind or another.

Bring on the burgers   They aren't as bad as you might think, despite their saturated fat. Ask for a whole-wheat bun and go easy on the special sauces, mayo topping, and slices of cheese. These can easily double the calorie load of a plain burger. Instead, stack it with veggie toppings: tomatoes, onions, lettuce, sprouts, or whatever's available.

Fear no fowl   You can lose weight, and stay a lot healthier, simply by ordering chicken instead of beef. As long as you don't have high blood pressure (since many chicken dishes are alarmingly high in salt), grilled chicken is among the healthiest items on the menu. The Sizzling Chicken Skillet at Applebee's, for example, has only 360 calories and 4 grams of fat.

Decoding the Menu

The biggest problem with eating away from home is that it's almost impossible to know exactly what's in each bite. Here are some reliable fat-and-calorie cues:

If the menu says: baked, broiled, charbroiled, grilled, steamed, stir-fried . . .

It means: These foods are cooked with relatively little added fats.

If the menu says: fried, alfredo, au gratin, pan-fried, "rich," or "with gravy" . . .

It means: Watch out, you're about to eat a fat bomb!

Eleven Questions to Ask the Waiter

Casual-dining restaurants are nothing like those sleek, haute cuisine emporiums staffed with waiters who apparently have nothing better to do than look down their noses when you ask for a translation of the French menu. The staff at chain restaurants such as Chili's and Applebee's are trained to take requests—and questions—seriously. Menus rarely give complete nutritional information or explain in detail how dishes are prepared. The waitstaff is there to help out, even if that means walking back to the kitchen and checking with the chef.

You're paying good money when you eat out. You deserve to know what you're getting—or to make reasonable changes to standard menu items. Here are some good questions to ask the waiter.

1. **"Is it okay if I substitute?"**   Just because the menu says the broiled chicken comes with fried potatoes doesn't mean it's written in stone. Most restaurants will happily substitute a leaner side dish for one that's higher in fat, such as steamed vegetables for potatoes, rice for cheese-covered beans, mustard for mayo on a sandwich, and salsa for sour cream on a baked potato.

2. **"How is it prepared"?**   You can tell a lot about the fat- and calorie-load of a dish just by knowing what the chef's up to. An entrée or side dish that's broiled, steamed, poached, boiled, baked, or stir-fried will almost always have less fat and calories than the same dish that's pan-fried or deep-fried.

3. **"Which cuts of meat do you use?"**   You'll already know the answer if you're ordering a steak, but there's no way to know about other beef dishes, such as a stir-fry, without asking. The difference can be significant. A lean cut of meat, such as tenderloin or sirloin, can have dramatically less fat than more succulent cuts, such as a skirt steak or brisket.

4. **"What kinds of oil do you use?"**   Calorie-wise, foods prepared with vegetable oils such as corn, canola, or safflower oil are not much better than those made with butter, cream, or lard. Olive oil is always the healthful choice. Don't be afraid to request it (after all, it's your heart)—and to go easy on it.

5. **"What's on it?"**   This is critical information if you're ordering a sandwich, or even a plate of steamed vegetables. They're almost always topped with something—mayo, rich cheese sauces, you name it. A steak supper often will have fewer calories than vegetables buried in a cheese sauce.

6. **"Can I have it 'light'?"**   That's restaurant code for "without (or with less) butter or oil." It doesn't apply to everything in the kitchen. It mainly refers to those items that get drenched with butter after cooking, such as steamed vegetables or grilled fish.

7. **"What does 'light' mean?"**   Many restaurants promote menu items with the word "light" (or sometimes "lite"). Does it mean light in flavor? Light in color? Or, as you'd

expect, lower in fat and calories? Don't assume that it's the latter. Ask.

8. **"Can we customize this?"**   You're the customer, so ask for things the way you want them. Most chefs are happy to oblige, as long as it doesn't take them any extra time or require more-expensive ingredients. If the menu offers a few higher-fat chicken breast dishes, for example, ask if the chef can simply broil a chicken breast and top it with tomato sauce. Or put together a plate of rice and vegetables.

9. **"How big is it?"**   Never assume that the serving sizes in restaurants even come close to approximating reasonable portions. Size really counts if you're ordering something labeled "low-fat." Federal guidelines require that an item advertised as low-fat have no more than 3 grams per serving. Sounds good, until you remember that the average restaurant portion might be three or four times the "official" serving size. So much for the "low-fat" claim. A four-ounce portion of steak gives you all the protein you need for a day, but most restaurants serve steaks up to three or four times that weight.

10. **"Can I have what she's having?"**   Here's another way to move beyond the menu basics. Suppose you see a melon salad on another diner's plate. You might not have a taste for salad, but that melon sure looks good. Ask the waiter if you can have a big slice for dessert. You'll probably get it.

11. **"Can you box it?"**   One of the joys of going to restaurants is that there's always something to take home for the next meal or snack. (Given the usual serving sizes, there *should* be leftovers.) Forget what your mom told you: you don't have to clean your plate. Eat a third, half, two-thirds, whatever—and have the waiter box up the rest. If you don't

trust your self-control, you can always ask the waiter to put half of your meal in a box even before it arrives on your plate.

Want more tips? For more dining-out tips like these, go to our free Web site at www.thefastfooddiet.com.

Pizza delivers   Here's some great news for those nights when you want to prop your feet up and eat in front of the TV. Pizza with a thin crust (whole wheat, if possible), light on the cheese and loaded with vegetable toppings, is a weight-loss meal in a box. Consider the Pizza Hut Thin 'N Crispy, with olives and mushrooms. One slice has only about 190 calories, with less than 4 grams of saturated fat.

New links in the restaurant chain   Just about every fast-food joint offers some healthy foods, but a few new chains have designed their menus entirely for healthy eating. Daily's Fit and Fresh, a chain based in San Diego, was the brainchild of a cardiac surgeon. Nothing on the menu contains more than 10 grams of fat. Other healthy chains include Fresh Choice, the Zone Café, and O'Naturals. P.F. Chang's has a surprisingly comprehensive vegetarian selection. Even Taco Bell offers tasty and inexpensive bean burritos and tacos. Request that they substitute guacamole and rice for the cheese and sour cream, and you'll be well off.

Trust yourself   This is really all you need to know to improve your eating habits so you'll lose weight and live longer. Making simple changes like these can also protect you from needing expensive prescription drugs to control such medical problems as high cholesterol, hypertension, and diabetes, among others. Remember, small changes in your eating habits can quickly add up to big improvements in your health. And you only need to be good 80 percent of the time.

CHAPTER 6

The Fast-Food Diet at the Mall

There's plenty of fast food in America's malls. And if you think the prices at those boutiques and department stores are a little rich, wait until you sample the snacks. There's as much hidden fat and calories lurking in those tempting muffins, pretzels, and ice-cream smoothies as in anything you'd order at a burger joint.

In most North American cities and towns, the shopping mall has taken the place of traditional downtown shopping. It's the place to take the family, stroll from shop to shop, and, of course, get some food at the expansive food courts. Downtown you actually had to walk from restaurant to restaurant, which burned a few extra calories. In the mall, nearly all of the calories are side-by-side or an escalator ride away. You can sample from a dozen or more menus without taking more than a few steps.

It's not impossible to integrate mall food into a nutritious weight-loss plan; it's just not easy. Mall restaurants are even less likely than fast-food chains to reveal the nutritional contents of their menu items, so you can never be entirely sure of what you're getting. But you can be pretty sure of one thing: these restaurants don't skimp on the fat or calories. Since you shouldn't assume that *anything* is good for you, I've done some homework for you here.

Au Bon Pain

This slightly upscale bakery-sandwich-salad shop is a fixture in malls as well as downtowns around the country. It offers a better selection of *lower-* (not necessarily low-) calorie items than you'll find in many of the other chains. Plus, there's a good selection of multigrain baked goods that provide ample amounts of fiber and low-glycemic carbs. Here are your best choices.

Honey Nine Grain Bagel   As long as you don't overload it with cream cheese (better, ask for the "lite" cream cheese, with one-third fewer calories), it can be a fine choice— nutritious enough to feel good about, and filling enough to get you through another hour's shopping. Vital stats: *360 calories, 2 grams total fat, 0 grams saturated fat.*

Low-Fat Triple Berry Muffin   This one isn't too bad, either, although the sugar content (31 grams) is on the high side. But who can say no to extra berries? Vital stats: *290 calories, 2 grams total fat, 0.5 grams saturated fat.*

Mediterranean Wrap   It's loaded with roasted red pepper, hummus, tomatoes, olives, and more. It's like eating a garden-fresh salad in a wrap! Vital stats: *571 calories, 22 grams total fat, 2.5 grams saturated fat.*

Spicy Tuna on Multigrain Bread   With healthful ingredients like this, you can't go very wrong. It's a little high on the calories, though, so you're best off ordering a half sandwich and enjoying it with a cup of soup. Vital stats: *690 calories, 33 grams total fat, 4 grams saturated fat.*

Dunkin' Donuts

Who expects to walk into any doughnut shop and walk out with a clear conscience? Doughnuts are usually fried in shortening that's loaded with trans fat, an artificially manufactured grease that researchers say is worse for your heart than saturated fats. Then there's the calorie load: just one doughnut can deliver as many calories as a sandwich—and a lot more fat. Is there anything in a Dunkin' Donuts that *won't* blow your diet? Not really. Here's the best you can do.

Multigrain Bagel with Low-Fat Cream Cheese   Nutrition, like life, is all about compromise. I'm not pretending this is a health food. It's not. But it's better than anything else on the menu, and the fat in the cream cheese will lessen the insulin response. Spread on only about one teaspoon's worth. Go for it if you must, but then cut back on fat calories elsewhere during the day. Vital stats: *540 calories, 22 grams total fat, 14 grams saturated fat.*

Sbarro

This may not be the best-tasting Italian food in the world, but it's far from the worst in terms of fat and calories. Just be aware that a single slice of certain pizzas at this chain can sink the best cardio-protection and diet plan, with about 500 calories and fat in the double digits. You can get something a little healthier—but just a little. Unfortunately, the company's Web site doesn't list the amount of saturated fat in their menu items. Here are the three healthiest picks you can choose.

Fresh Tomato Pizza   It's at the restaurant's low end of fat-and-calorie content, and generous helpings of tomato are always good. Vital stats per slice: *450 calories, 14 grams total fat.*

Low-Carb Pepperoni Pizza   I'm not impressed with anything that's labeled "low-carb," but that's a personal bias. This pizza actually ranks pretty well on the fat and calorie scale. Vital stats per slice: *420 calories, 14 grams total fat.*

Pasta Primavera Salad   It's more filling than a basic green salad, and lean enough to enjoy without feeling guilty. Go easy on the dressing! Vital stats: *190 calories, 10 grams total fat.*

Panda Express

Naturally, it's a challenge to get vegetables at any of the fast-food chains, unless you count the pickles, onions, and toma-toes. But at Panda Express, you can order rice or noodle dishes heaped with greens, which is just what you want when you're eating for your weight and your health. Try these six top picks.

Mixed Vegetables   Combined with the steamed rice, this is a wholesome meal that will kick up your vegetable consump-tion toward the levels recommended for lowering choles-terol and reducing the risk of heart disease and cancer. Vital stats: *70 calories, 3 grams total fat, 0.5 grams saturated fat.*

Steamed Rice   Because it's white rice rather than brown, it's not as good for weight loss as a lower-glycemic carb would be. But it's still better than a doughnut—and it rounds out other meals on the menu. Vital stats: *330 calories, 0.5 grams total fat, 0 grams saturated fat.*

Beef with String Beans   A little protein and a little vegetable— not bad for a light meal. Vital stats: *170 calories, 9 grams total fat, 2 grams saturated fat.*

Spicy Chicken with Peanuts   You already know that chicken is a good substitute for beef—but did you know that people who eat nuts and legumes tend to be healthier than those who don't? It's a medical fact! Vital stats: *200 calories, 7 grams total fat, 1.5 grams saturated fat.*

String Beans with Fried Tofu   I rarely recommend any kind of fried food, but this one isn't too bad. And let's face it, frying tofu makes it taste better than steaming it. Vital stats: *180 calories, 11 grams total fat, 2 grams saturated fat.*

Vegetables with Fried Rice   Again, frying kicks up the fat in this dish higher than I'd like to see it, but the saturated-fat content is low, and the extra vegetable serving makes it money well spent. Vital stats: *390 calories, 12 grams total fat, 2.5 grams saturated fat.*

Schlotzsky's

Eating a traditional submarine sandwich made with whole-grain bread, piled with fresh vegetables, and flavored with a drizzle of olive oil is like having the best weight-loss elements of my diet on a roll. But size does count—and at Schlotzsky's "big" can be really big, with some sandwiches packing more than 1,000 calories and enormous amounts of fat. As long as you order something more modestly scaled, you can have a nutritious, filling lunch that won't bust the diet bank. Try either of these.

Dijon Grilled Chicken Sandwich   Many fast-food chicken entrées are jammed with salt—nearly an entire day's worth in one serving. Fortunately, this sandwich isn't—and it's low enough in calories and fat to eat every day and lose weight. Vital stats: *330 calories, 4 grams total fat, 1 gram saturated fat.*

Turkey & Guacamole   Avocados are about the only fruit that contain an appreciable amount of fat (in this case, nearly 70 percent). That's a lot of extra calories if you're one of those people who can eat an entire avocado at one meal. But their fat is mainly the healthy, monounsaturated kind—and there isn't enough avocado on this sandwich to make the extra calories a significant concern. Vital stats: *450 calories, 15 grams total fat, 2 grams saturated fat.*

Smoothies and Juices

I often advise my patients to start the day with a glass of fresh-squeezed juice or a fruit smoothie. It's an easy way to add a few extra fruit servings to your daily diet. Fruit is an integral part of a good weight-loss plan because most is low in calories and high in fiber and antioxidants. If you make a smoothie with soy milk, you're also getting *isoflavones*, soy compounds that are great for the heart and bones. The FDA recently gave food manufacturers permission to put health labels on products high in soy protein, indicating that they can help lower heart disease risk. Even if you make a smoothie with skim milk, you're getting a good blast of protein, which is ideal for satisfying your appetite between meals, without the fat.

It's hard to go wrong with juices and smoothies, but of course the food court chains have managed to do it. Many of their drinks are jammed with so much sugar that it can spike your insulin—and the resulting fat storage—into the danger zone. Worse, many of these drinks are enormous, with up to 40 ounces per serving, and some mix the fruit with ice cream, driving up the fat and calorie content. No mistake about it: drink one every day and you're going to gain weight. These drinks are often closer to a dessert than a healthful beverage, so munching a handful of mixed nuts as you sip will help balance the sugar and control your appetite later on. You may certainly enjoy them—but check the nutritional information first.

Jamba Juice

This chain is known for its fresh-squeezed juices, "enlightened smoothies," and so-called boosts that add valuable nutrients yet few calories to their drinks. We recommend these.

Orange/Carrot Juice, 16-ounce   A blend of 100 percent pure fresh-squeezed orange and carrot juices—it doesn't get any healthier. Vital stats: *160 calories, 1 gram total fat, 0 grams saturated fat.*

Passion Berry Breeze, 16-ounce   This is a choice from the Enlightened Smoothies menu using a lower-calorie dairy base blended with passion fruit juice, mangoes, strawberries, and peaches—delicious. Vital stats: *150 calories, 0 grams total fat, 0 grams saturated fat.*

Mango Mantra, 16-ounce   This smoothie is not only low in calories because of its lower-calorie dairy base, but also high in vitamin C thanks to 100 percent pure orange juice used along with mangos and peaches. Vital stats: *170 calories, 0.5 grams total fat, 0 grams saturated fat.*

Tropical Awakening, 16-ounce   Here blueberries, which are high in antioxidants, are blended with tropical pineapple and bananas and the reduced-calorie base. Vital stats: *190 calories, 0.5 grams total fat, 0 grams saturated fat.*

TCBY

This chain sells soft-frozen yogurt as well as smoothies. The word "yogurt" is almost synonymous with good health, but don't let it fool you into thinking that everything on the menu is good for weight loss. It isn't. Still, there are some good picks.

Berry Slim without Yogurt, 20-ounce   It isn't exactly a low-calorie drink, but if you think of it as dessert, the slightly high calorie load is easier to forgive. Vital stats: *300 calories, 0 grams total fat, 0 grams saturated fat.*

No-Sugar-Added Nonfat Frozen Yogurt, 4-ounce   If you like yogurt and can do without the rich "mouth feel" of higher-fat desserts, this is as lean as it gets. Enjoy! Vital stats: *90 calories, 0 grams total fat, 0 grams saturated fat.*

Raspberry De-lite without Yogurt, 20-ounce   This is one of the best smoothies you can buy—low in calories, loaded with protective antioxidants, and delicious. Vital stats: *240 calories, 0 grams total fat, 0 grams saturated fat.*

Tropical Replenisher without Yogurt, 20-ounce   When you're watching your weight, you'll smile after you polish off one of these. It's one of the tastiest drinks out there and won't make a dent in your diet—assuming, of course, you don't load up on calories the rest of the day. Vital stats: *240 calories, 0 grams total fat, 0 grams saturated fat.*

Orange Julius

This chain is renowned for its deliciously frothy drinks. They're certainly lean enough to have every day, but don't confuse them with "straight" fruit juice. They're quite a bit richer than that. You'll be fine if you stick to the 16-ounce size. Or better, split one with a friend. Try one of these.

Orange Julius, 16-ounce   This flagship product is what put the chain on the food-court map. Vital stats: *220 calories, 1 gram total fat, 0 grams saturated fat*. The strawberry drink clocks in at the same calorie-and-fat content.

Muscle Peach Smoothie, 20-ounce   It's made with nonfat vanilla frozen yogurt in addition to fruit so you'll get a healthy dose of calcium, too. Vital stats: *260 calories, 0.5 grams total fat, 0 grams saturated fat*.

CHAPTER 7

The Six-Week Fast-Food Diet

L et's say you are someone who is on the run from dawn till the late night. You have absolutely no time to cook for yourself. How can you eat healthily and lose weight on your hectic schedule? You'll find the answer in the next pages. It's a no-brainer weight-loss plan for eating out all the time. Note that most of the daily menus weigh in around 1,500 calories; that's what the average woman should eat if she wants to stop gaining weight and start losing it. If you're a guy, bump it up to around 1,800 calories a day. Regarding beverages: Soft drinks, sodas, and even diet sodas should be avoided as much as possible. All trigger weight gain. If you must have a soda, make it a spritzer— a soda diluted with one-half carbonated water. Other acceptable beverages include carbonated water with lemon, plain water, coffee or tea (hot or iced or espresso) either unsweetened or with stevia or nonfat or low-fat milk.

By the end of the six weeks, you should be 10 to 15 pounds lighter. Add my walking plan (see chapter 14) and you'll lose even more.

You'll notice that the diet plan covers Mondays through Fridays. This is to encourage you to tackle the task of healthful yet easy home-cooking on the remaining two days—which don't have to be the weekend, of course, if you'd rather preserve time for other activities then. Armed with your new knowledge, you'll be able to serve nutritious and delicious meals to your family. Chapter 8 includes many recipes as well as shopping and cooking tips for you to try out to keep your time in the kitchen short and stress free. Appendix B offers a varied selection of healthful snacks for the little appetite in between. And best, log onto our free Web site, www.thefastfooddiet.com, to find even more, frequently updated recipes and tips. Bon appetit!

WEEK 1: MONDAY

Meal	Restaurant	Food	Calories	Fat (grams)
Breakfast	Arby's	Breakfast Sourdough Sandwich with Egg & Cheese	330	16
Midmorning snack	Convenience store	Small mixed fruit	70	0
		Stonyfield Organic Low-fat Yogurt (small container)	140	1.5
Lunch	McDonald's	Caesar Salad with Grilled Chicken	220	6
		Fruit 'n Yogurt Parfait	160	2
Midafternoon snack	From home	Banana (1)	105	0
		Walnuts (1 handful)	175	17
Supper	Boston Market	Double-Sauced Angus Meat Loaf	310	19
		Garlic Dill New Potatoes	130	2.5
		Green Beans	70	4
Totals			**1,710**	**68**

WEEK 1: TUESDAY

Meal	Restaurant	Food	Calories	Fat (grams)
Breakfast	Burger King	French Toast Sticks (5)	390	20
Midmorning snack	Convenience store	Macadamia nuts ($^1/_2$ oz.) or 1 pear	190	10
Lunch	Del Taco	Chicken Soft Taco	210	12
		Beans 'n Cheese Cup	260	3
Midafternoon snack	From home	Apple	72	0
		Cheddar cheese (1-oz. cube)	114	9
Supper	Papa John's	Original Crust Pizza, Spinach Alfredo Chicken Tomato (14-inch—1 slice)	200	7
		Side Salad with Low-fat Dressing	138	4.2
Totals			**1,574**	**65.2**

WEEK 1: WEDNESDAY

Meal	Restaurant	Food	Calories	Fat (grams)
Breakfast	Dunkin' Donuts	Multigrain Bagel with Low-fat Cream Cheese	450	10
Midmorning snack	Convenience store	Stonyfield Organic Low-fat Yogurt (small container)	140	1.5
		Apple or pear	72	0
Lunch	KFC	Tender Roast Chicken Sandwich with Sauce	400	19
Midafternoon snack	Vending machine	Roasted peanuts (1 oz.)	160	14
Supper	Panda Express	Veggie Spring Roll	80	2.5
		Beef with Broccoli (marinated beef and broccoli stir-fried in an oyster-based soy sauce)	150	8
Totals			**1,452**	**55**

WEEK 1: THURSDAY

Meal	Restaurant	Food	Calories	Fat (grams)
Breakfast	McDonald's	Bacon, Egg and Cheese McGriddles	450	23
Midmorning snack	From home	Apple or pear Mixed nuts (1 tbsp.)	72 197	0 14
Lunch	Olive Garden	Linguine alla Marinara (tomatoes, onions, herbs on pasta) Side Salad with Nonfat Dressing	316 120	5 0
Midafternoon snack	From home	Homemade granola with nuts (1 handful)	150	8
Supper	Denny's	Carb-Watch Grilled Chicken Dinner Side Garden Salad with Fat-free Ranch Dressing	315 138	8 4
Totals			**1,758**	**62**

WEEK 1: FRIDAY

Meal	Restaurant	Food	Calories	Fat (grams)
Breakfast	Arby's	Biscuit with Ham	270	13
Midmorning snack	From home	Grapes (1 bunch)	110	0
Lunch	Baja Fresh Mexican Grill	Taco Chilito with Chicken Wild Gulf Shrimp Side Salad	260 150 70	9 2 3
Midafternoon snack	From home	1 celery stick and 1 hard-boiled egg	105	8
Supper	Bob Evans	Catfish, Grilled New Orleans Style Baked Potato, Plain Specialty Side Salad (no croutons)	255 207 115	19 0 7
Totals			**1,542**	**61**

WEEK 2: MONDAY

Meal	Restaurant	Food	Calories	Fat (grams)
Breakfast	Hardee's	Frisco Breakfast Sandwich	410	17
Midmorning snack	Supermarket	Almonds (1 handful)	207	18
Lunch	Burger King	Original Whopper Jr. Sandwich (without mayo)	310	13
		Side Garden Salad with Fat-free Dressing	60	0
Midafternoon snack	Vending machine	Handful of dried fruit and nuts (about 1 1/2 oz.)	180	8
Supper	Church's Chicken	Fried Chicken Breast	200	12.5
		Corn on the Cob	140	3
		Mashed Potatoes	90	3.5
Totals			**1,597**	**75**

WEEK 2: TUESDAY

Meal	Restaurant	Food	Calories	Fat (grams)
Breakfast	Del Taco	Breakfast Burrito	250	11
Midmorning snack	Vending machine	Roasted peanuts/ almonds (1 oz.)	160	14
Lunch	Pizza Hut	Full House Extra-Large Pizza, Veggie Lover's (16-inch—1 slice)	260	11
		Side Salad with Low-fat Dressing	130	0
Midafternoon snack	Convenience store	Handful of dried fruit and nuts (about 1 1/2 oz.)	180	8
Supper	Golden Corral	Pork Chop or Loin Slices, Grilled	120	4
		Timberline Chili, Cup	280	13
		Cornbread (skillet)	85	2
		Broccoli, Steamed	25	0
Totals			**1,490**	**63**

WEEK 2: WEDNESDAY

Meal	Restaurant	Food	Calories	Fat (grams)
Breakfast	Hardee's	Scrambled Eggs	160	12
		Pancakes (3)	300	5
Midmorning snack	Health food store	Balance Bar	200	6
Lunch	Jack in the Box	Grilled Chicken Fillet Sandwich	430	19
Midafternoon snack	McDonald's	Fruit 'n Yogurt Parfait	160	2
Supper	P.F. Chang's China Bistro	Cantonese Shrimp (stir-fried with garlic, chives, and snow peas)	370	13
		Sichuan-Style Asparagus (stir-fried with Sichuan vegetables)	110	3.5
Totals			**1,730**	**60.5**

WEEK 2: THURSDAY

Meal	Restaurant	Food	Calories	Fat (grams)
Breakfast	McDonald's	Egg McMuffin	300	12
Midmorning snack	Supermarket	Trail Mix (1 oz.)	194	12
Lunch	KFC	Tender Roast Chicken Sandwich (without skin)	169	4.3
		Corn on the Cob (3-inch)	90	0.5
		Mean Greens	70	3
Midafternoon snack	Panera Bread	Half of a Blueberry Bagel with Low-fat Cream Cheese	290	4.5
Supper	Olive Garden	Capellini Pomodoro (tomatoes, garlic, fresh basil, and extra-virgin olive oil tossed with capellini)	387	9

Meal	Restaurant	Food	Calories	Fat (grams)
Supper cont'd.		Broiled Salmon (small side portion—4 oz.)	220	10
		Side Salad with Nonfat Dressing	120	0
Totals			**1,840**	**55**

WEEK 2: FRIDAY

Meal	Restaurant	Food	Calories	Fat (grams)
Breakfast	Arby's	Scrambled Egg	80	6
		Potato Cakes	250	15
Midmorning snack	Dunkin' Donuts	1/2 Multigrain Bagel with Low-fat Cream Cheese	225	5
Lunch	Subway	Veggie Delite (6-inch sub with lettuce, tomatoes, red onions, green peppers, olives, and pickles on whole-wheat bun)	230	3
		Double Chocolate Chip Cookie	210	10
Midafternoon snack	Convenience store	Stonyfield Organic Low-fat Yogurt (small container)	140	1.5
		Roasted peanuts (1 oz.)	160	14
Supper	Wendy's	Mandarin Chicken Salad (iceberg, romaine, spring salad mix, mandarin oranges, diced chicken)	150	1.5
		Fat-free French Dressing	80	0
Totals			**1,525**	**56**

WEEK 3: MONDAY

Meal	Restaurant	Food	Calories	Fat (grams)
Breakfast	Home	Bowl of Shredded Wheat Cereal with skim milk and 1/2 sliced banana or handful of blueberries or raspberries	371	1
Midmorning snack	TCBY	Tropical Replenisher Smoothie	240	0
Lunch	Hardee's	Roast Beef Sandwich (regular size)	330	16
		Coleslaw (small order)	240	20
Midafternoon snack	From home	Homemade granola (1 handful)	150	8
Supper	Bojangles	Southern Style Chicken Breast (1 pc.)	260	16
		Potatoes without Gravy	80	1
		Corn on the Cob	140	2
Totals			**1,811**	**64**

WEEK 3: TUESDAY

Meal	Restaurant	Food	Calories	Fat (grams)
Breakfast	Bruegger's	Atlantic Smoked Salmon Bagel Sandwich	470	12
Midmorning snack	From home	Apple	72	0
		Stonyfield Organic Low-fat Yogurt (small container)	140	1.5
Lunch	Burger King	BK Veggie Burger (without mayo)	300	7
		Chicken Tenders (4 pcs.)	170	9
Midafternoon snack	Convenience store	Walnuts or Almonds (1 handful)	175	17
Supper	Baja Fresh Mexican Grill	Charbroiled Fish	210	3
		Baja Fresh Mex-Grill Rice	280	4
		Fresh Guacamole (3-oz. side)	110	13
Totals			**1,927**	**66.5**

WEEK 3: WEDNESDAY

Meal	Restaurant	Food	Calories	Fat (grams)
Breakfast	Bob Evans	Scrambled Eggs	170	11
		Canadian Bacon	20	1
		Home Fries	150	2
		Half of an English Muffin	70	1
Midmorning snack	Convenience store	Stonyfield Organic Smoothie Style Yogurt (small container)	150	2
Lunch	Wendy's	Hot Stuffed Baked Potato Topped with Chili (small)	510	6
Midafternoon snack	Convenience store	Part-skim mozzarella cheese stick	70	4
Supper	Boston Market	Smokehouse BBQ Grilled Chicken	370	12
		Creamed Spinach	200	17
		Steamed Vegetable Medley	30	0
Totals			**1,740**	**56**

WEEK 3: THURSDAY

Meal	Restaurant	Food	Calories	Fat (grams)
Breakfast	Chick-fil-A	Fresh Fruit Cup, Large	100	0.5
		Breakfast Item—Biscuit with Egg	340	16
Midmorning snack	From home	Homemade granola (1 handful)	150	8
Lunch	Dairy Queen	BBQ Beef Sandwich	300	9
		Side Salad	60	2.5
		Fudge Bar (non-fat)	50	0
Midafternoon snack	Convenience store	Macadamia nuts ($^{1}/_{2}$ oz.)	110	10
Supper	Olive Garden	Ministrone Soup	100	1
		Shrimp Primavera	630	13
		Garden Salad with Low-fat Italian Dressing	50	2
Totals			**1,890**	**62**

WEEK 3: FRIDAY

Meal	Restaurant	Food	Calories	Fat (grams)
Breakfast	Denny's	Oatmeal N' Fixins	460	6
		Honeydew Melon	30	0
Midmorning snack	From home	Grapes (1 bunch)	110	0
Lunch	Wendy's	Small Chili	330	9
		Side Salad	35	0
Midafternoon snack	Convenience store	Swiss Amish cheese (1 oz.)	91	6
		Apple	72	0
Supper	El Pollo Loco	Taco Al Carbon	135	3
		Pinto Beans	155	4
		Coleslaw	205	16
Totals			**1,623**	**44**

WEEK 4: MONDAY

Meal	Restaurant	Food	Calories	Fat (grams)
Breakfast	Golden Corral	Scrambled Eggs	160	10
		Hash Browns	100	7
Midmorning snack	Convenience store	Stonyfield Organic Low-fat Yogurt (small container)	140	0.5
Lunch	Subway	Roasted Chicken Breast Salad (roasted chicken breast, lettuce, tomatoes, onions, green peppers, olives, and pickles)	140	3
		Fat-free Red Wine Vinaigrette	30	0.3
		Minestrone Soup	70	1
		White Macadamia Nut Cookie	210	11
Midafternoon snack	Convenience store	Apple	82	0

Meal	Restaurant	Food	Calories	Fat (grams)
Supper	Chipotle	Grilled Steak	230	12
		Fajita Vegetables	100	8
		Black Beans	130	1
Totals			**1,392**	**53.8**

WEEK 4: TUESDAY

Meal	Restaurant	Food	Calories	Fat (grams)
Breakfast	McDonald's	Egg McMuffin	300	12
Midmorning snack	Convenience store	Apple	72	0
Lunch	Olive Garden	Chicken Giardino (fresh vegetables and chicken with farfalle pasta in a lemon-herb sauce)	447	14.5
		Side Salad with Non-fat Dressing	120	0
Midafternoon snack	Orange Julius	Orange Julius (16 oz.)	220	1
Supper	Bob Evans	Catfish, Grilled New Orleans Style	255	19
		Baked Potato, Plain	207	0
		Specialty Side Salad (no croutons)	115.7	0
Totals			**1,736.7**	**46.5**

WEEK 4: WEDNESDAY

Meal	Restaurant	Food	Calories	Fat (grams)
Breakfast	Bruegger's	Honey-Grain Bagel	330	3
		Cream Cheese, Light Strawberry	70	4
Midmorning snack	Supermarket	Trail mix	194	12
Lunch	Carl's Jr.	Hamburger	280	9
		Garden Salad-to-Go	120	3

Meal	Restaurant	Food	Calories	Fat (grams)
Midafternoon snack	Health food store	Think Organic Fruit and Nut Snack Bar	190	9
Supper	Red Lobster	Lobster Chops (3 grilled skewers with a split Maine lobster tail wrapped around a jumbo sea scallop)	321	9
		Baked Potato	130	0
		Garden Salad	50	1
		Fat-free Ranch Dressing	50	0
Totals			**1,735**	**50**

WEEK 4: THURSDAY

Meal	Restaurant	Food	Calories	Fat (grams)
Breakfast	Carl's Jr.	Sourdough Breakfast Sandwich with Ham	450	20
Midmorning snack	From home	Walnuts (1 handful)	175	17
Lunch	Subway	Turkey Sub (6-inch with lettuce and tomato on a whole-wheat bun)	280	5
		Minestrone Soup	89	1
Midafternoon snack	From home	Banana (1)	105	0
Supper	Golden Corral	Meat Loaf	190	10
		Tomato Pasta Florentine Soup	90	1.5
		Mashed Potatoes	120	6
		Green Peas	110	5
Totals			**1,609**	**65.5**

WEEK 4: FRIDAY

Meal	Restaurant	Food	Calories	Fat (grams)
Breakfast	Jack in the Box	Breakfast Jack Sandwich	310	14
		Hash Browns	150	10
Midmorning snack	Convenience store	Fresh fruit cup	139	0
Lunch	McDonald's	Hot 'n Spicy McChicken Sandwich (without mayo)	330	12
		French Fries (small)	210	10
Midafternoon snack	TCBY	Tropical Replenisher Smoothie	240	0
Supper	Red Lobster	Jumbo Shrimp Cocktail Dinner	228	4
		Baked Potato	103	0
		Garden Salad	50	1
		Fat-free Ranch Dressing	50	0
Totals			**1,810**	**51**

WEEK 5: MONDAY

Meal	Restaurant	Food	Calories	Fat (grams)
Breakfast	Bob Evans	Eggs, Over Easy	93	7
		Bacon	36	4
		Grits	150	7
		French Toast	135	2
Midmorning snack	Panera Bread	Half of a Multigrain Bagel with Low-fat Cream Cheese	290	4.5
Lunch	Wahoo's Fish Taco	Taco with Fish of the Day (flamebroiled or blackened fish)	225.6	4.6
		Beans (side order—stewed with herbs and spices, no added oil)	313.5	1.2
Midafternoon snack	Convenience store	Swiss Amish cheese (1 oz.)	91	6
		Apple	72	0
Supper	Panda Express	Black Pepper Chicken (spicy)	180	10
		Vegetable Chow Mein	330	11
Totals			**1,916.1**	**57.3**

WEEK 5: TUESDAY

Meal	Restaurant	Food	Calories	Fat (grams)
Breakfast	Arby's	Sourdough Egg 'n Cheese	330	16
Midmorning snack	From home	Blueberries or raspberries (1 handful)	105	0
		Stonyfield Organic Low-fat Yogurt (small container)	140	0.5
Lunch	McDonald's	Grilled Chicken Flatbread Sandwich (without cheese)	390	12
		Fruit 'n Yogurt Parfait (without granola)	130	2
Midafternoon snack	From home	Macadamia nuts or walnuts ($^1/_2$ oz.)	190	10
Supper	Red Lobster	Bayou Style Seafood Gumbo (6 oz.)	120	4
		Live Maine Lobster, Steamed (1.25 lb.)	160	1
		Garden Salad	50	1
		Fat-free Ranch Dressing	50	0
Totals			**1,665**	**46.5**

WEEK 5: WEDNESDAY

Meal	Restaurant	Food	Calories	Fat (grams)
Breakfast	McDonald's	Bacon, Egg, and Cheese Biscuit	440	24
Midmorning snack	Convenience store	Stonyfield Organic Smoothie Style Yogurt (small container)	150	2
Lunch	Wendy's	Chili (small)	200	6
		Jr. Hamburger (2-oz. beef patty, ketchup, mustard, dill pickles, onion, sandwich bun)	300	7

Meal	Restaurant	Food	Calories	Fat (grams)
Midafternoon snack	From home	Celery sticks and 1 hard-boiled egg	105	8
Supper	Long John Silver's	Flavorbaked Fish & Chicken Combination (1 pc. each, over rice with baked potato and green beans)	538	10
Totals			**1,733**	**57**

WEEK 5: THURSDAY

Meal	Restaurant	Food	Calories	Fat (grams)
Breakfast	Carl's Jr.	Croissant Sunrise Sandwich, No Meat	360	21
Midmorning snack	Supermarket	Handful of Trail Mix (about 1–2 oz.)	194	10
Lunch	Panera Bread	Corn & Green Chili Chowder	190	8
		Half of a Chicken Salad Sandwich on Nine Grain Bread (chicken salad made with all white meat, mayo, spicy mustard, lettuce, tomatoes, red onions, sprouts, and salt and pepper)	320	14.5
Midafternoon snack	From home	Stonyfield Organic Low-fat Yogurt (small container)	140	1.5
Supper	P.F. Chang's China Bistro	Cantonese Scallops (stir-fried with garlic, chives, and snow peas)	370	13
		Spinach Stir-Fried with Garlic	110	3.5
Totals			**1,684**	**71.5**

WEEK 5: FRIDAY

Meal	Restaurant	Food	Calories	Fat (grams)
Breakfast	Burger King	French Toast Sticks (5)	390	20
Midmorning snack	Vending machine	Mixed dried fruit and nuts	180	8
Lunch	Wendy's	Chili (small)	200	6
		Grilled Chicken Sandwich (grilled chicken fillet, low-cal honey mustard dressing, tomato, lettuce, sandwich bun)	300	7
Midafternoon snack	Panera Bread	Half of a Blueberry Bagel with Low-fat Cream Cheese	290	4.5
Supper	Schlotzsky's Deli	Fresh Tomato & Pesto Pizza (8-inch—herbed sourdough crust, basil pesto, fresh tomato, onion, and mozzarella cheese)	539	16
		Small Garden Salad with Fat-free Dressing	23	1
Totals			**1,922**	**62.5**

WEEK 6: MONDAY

Meal	Restaurant	Food	Calories	Fat (grams)
Breakfast	Dunkin' Donuts	Multigrain Bagel with Low-fat Cream Cheese	450	10
Midmorning snack	From home	Apple	72	0
Lunch	Taco Bell	Burrito Supreme Chicken	410	16
		Salsa	27	0
Midafternoon snack	Convenience store	Macadamia nuts or walnuts ($^1/_2$ oz.)	190	10

Meal	Restaurant	Food	Calories	Fat (grams)
Supper	Schlotzsky's Deli	Mediterranean Pizza (8-inch—herbed sourdough crust, feta cheese, black olives, tomato, onion, basil pesto, and mozzarella cheese)	524	18
		Small Garden Salad with Fat-free Dressing	23	1
Totals			**1,696**	**55**

WEEK 6: TUESDAY

Meal	Restaurant	Food	Calories	Fat (grams)
Breakfast	Denny's	One Egg	120	10
		Hash Browns	220	14
		Dry Toast	90	1
		Cantaloupe Melon	30	0
Midmorning snack	Orange Julius	Orange Julius (16 oz.)	220	1
Lunch	Subway	Roasted Chicken Noodle Soup	90	4
		Sweet Onion Chicken Teriyaki Sub (6-inch Select Sub—teriyaki glazed chicken strips, lettuce, tomatoes, onions, green peppers, olives, and fat-free sweet onion select sauce on whole-wheat bun)	380	5
Midafternoon snack	Vending machine	Mixed dry fruit and nuts	160	6
Supper	Chipotle	Steak, Grilled	230	12
		Fajita Vegetables	100	8
		Black Beans	130	1
Totals			**1,770**	**62**

WEEK 6: WEDNESDAY

Meal	Restaurant	Food	Calories	Fat (grams)
Breakfast	Dunkin' Donuts	Biscuit, Egg & Cheese Sandwich	380	22
Midmorning snack	Vending machine	Roasted peanuts/almonds (1 oz.)	160	14
Lunch	Long John Silver	Flavorbaked Chicken (1 pc. over rice with baked potato and green beans)	448	7.5
Midafternoon snack	Convenience store	Stonyfield Organic Low-fat Yogurt (small container)	140	1.5
Supper	Wahoo's Fish Taco	Wahoo's Salad with Fish of the Day (flamebroiled or blackened fish)	573	29
Totals			**1,701**	**74**

WEEK 6: THURSDAY

Meal	Restaurant	Food	Calories	Fat (grams)
Breakfast	Denny's	Oatmeal N' Fixins (oatmeal, milk, raisins, sliced banana, choice of bread, and a glass of juice)	460	6
Midmorning snack	From home	Apple or pear	72	0
		Mixed nuts (1 tbsp.)	197	14
Lunch	Schlotzsky's Deli	Chicken Breast Sandwich (small size—sliced roasted chicken breast on a toasted sourdough bun with fat-free spicy ranch dressing, lettuce, tomato, and pickle slices)	337	3
		Beef & Black Bean Soup	150	1
Midafternoon snack	From home	Grapes (1 bunch)	110	0

Meal	Restaurant	Food	Calories	Fat (grams)
Supper	Golden Corral	Fish Fillet, Cajun Style	210	9.5
		Chicken Gumbo Soup	70	1.5
		Baked Potato, Plain	110	0
		Carrot & Raisin Salad	110	5
Totals			**1,826**	**40**

WEEK 6: FRIDAY

Meal	Restaurant	Food	Calories	Fat (grams)
Breakfast	Einstein Bros. Bagels	Honey Whole Wheat Bagel	320	1
		Whipped Honey Almond Cream Cheese, Reduced Fat	70	5
Midmorning snack	From home	Banana	105	0
Lunch	P.F. Chang's China Bistro	Steamed Shrimp Dumplings	320	12
		Buddha's Feast Steamed Mixed Vegetables	225	15
Midafternoon snack	Supermarket	Handful of Trail Mix (1–2 oz.)	194	12
Supper	Wendy's	Mediterranean Chicken Salad (iceberg, romaine and spring salad mix, Mediterranean herb—seasoned diced chicken, feta cheese, grape tomatoes, cucumbers, and red onion rings)	280	12
		Fat-free French Dressing	80	0
Totals			**1,594**	**57**

CHAPTER 8

Fast Food at Home

It's hard to argue with the appeal of the fast-food drive-thru lane. When your brain has turned to mush at the end of the day and there's a hungry six-year-old in the backseat on the verge of a tantrum, the idea of a kind stranger passing a ready-made hot meal through your car window is supremely inviting.

But we do not live by fast food alone. Thank goodness we get the occasional opportunity to enjoy a nutritious home-cooked meal with our families. Not only are these times great for family bonding, but they represent opportunities to enjoy some of the health-building, disease-fighting foods we miss when we eat fast food so often.

Home-cooked meals trigger healing on many levels. For one thing, you'll almost surely eat fewer calories. Home cooking is also cheaper than eating out. Sure, this book is showing you how to find low-cal chow at fast-food chains, but you can't always trust that you'll order that way when your energy is shot, your blood sugar's low, and all you want is to collapse onto the sofa. Besides, by the time you've pulled into the restaurant you're looking for and inhaled clouds of exhaust in the drive-up line, you might have already blown the "fast" part of the equation. You can move more quickly than that at home—providing you've prepared by shopping wisely.

A bare pantry and an empty fridge almost force you to veer off your diet. To avoid this, you've got to stock up ahead of time and have enough healthy foods on hand when you need to eat. A trip to the grocery store while ravenous is never a good idea. Few of us have the willpower to walk past all those seductive sights and smells when we're really hungry unless you're Superwoman or Superman. So don't do this to yourself.

What's in Your Kitchen

Browse through any cookbook and you're sure to find a few dozen calorie-smart recipes that you can prepare, beginning to end, in about ten minutes. The key is to have a ready supply of basic and versatile ingredients, the ones that go into just about every recipe. You also want to keep your pantry and fridge well stocked with "quick" ingredients that need a minimum of preparation. Those should be as nutritious as possible. Why? Because when you're hungry *everything* tastes good, so why not use this powerful urge to your advantage? Here are some tips to help you keep lots of reliable, low-calorie standbys on hand.

Load up on "instants" Canned beans, canned tuna, and ready-to-serve soups are the dietary equivalents of duct tape: You can use them for just about anything, anytime. No preparation required. Just open and use. For instance, while defrosting a chicken breast in the microwave and preheating the oven, open and combine a can of vegetables with a can of low-fat mushroom soup. Put the chicken breast in a casserole, cover with the vegetables and soup, and heat in the oven. Just throw a salad together and you're done, in about the same time you'd spend on a take-out order.

Let someone else do the chopping   Despite the claims of some recent trendy diets, no one lives on meat alone (not for long, anyway). Vegetables and salad greens are the mainstay of any effective weight-loss plan. Unfortunately, they take forever to prepare! Why waste time hauling out your knives and cutting board? These days, every supermarket provides a lot of shelf space for precut vegetables and salad mixes. Sure, they cost a little extra—but they're worth it for the time they'll save you.

Grab a cold one   You can't go wrong with frozen vegetables. They're just as nutritious and tasty as fresh ones and sometimes more so because they tend to be picked at the height of their season when flavors are peaking and then are frozen quickly. If you want to save even more time, buy your frozen veggies in single-serve, microwaveable pouches. That's one less pot you'll have to wash. Of course, you'll want to avoid frozen vegetables mixed in cream or butter sauces. Many of these products are delicious, but they can jam your diet with extra fat and calories that you don't really need.

Season without salt   Many fast-food and restaurant meals contain boatloads of salt. Studies show that most people can easily lower their blood pressure by 20 points or more— enough to avoid the need for medication in some cases—by limiting their daily salt intake to 1,500 milligrams or less. So put the shaker aside. Instead, season your food with herbs and spices such as black pepper, oregano, basil, and anything else you like. The next time you're at the supermarket, check out their selection of hot sauces, curries, or other international spices for exotic flavors. Just be sure to check the fat and salt content on the label before you drop them into your shopping cart. Once you get used to not using salt, highly salted foods will taste unpleasant to you.

Stock up on grains　They can really help you lose weight quickly because they are bulky yet contain few calories. They also control the rush of insulin into your bloodstream. The only problem with whole grains is they take time to cook—up to 60 minutes for brown rice or wheat berries, for example. Even refined white rice takes about 20 minutes. That's too long when you want something fast. However, small grains such as quinoa, amaranth, and millet need far less time—as little as 10 to 12 minutes—and they are not refined. Here's a clever shortcut: When you have a little extra time, cook up five or six cups of quinoa, brown rice, or any other whole grain. Use what you need for that night's meal and refrigerate or freeze the rest. Grains absorb water even after the initial cooking, so they'll remain firm and tender when you use them later. Another trick: Buy yourself a rice cooker and learn how to use it.

Load the freezer, load the fridge　You won't get very far with most quick recipes unless you have some ready-to-go protein. Good examples include one-percent milk, low-fat cheese, frozen chicken breasts, frozen shrimp, organic tofu, and lean beef. Don't try to skimp on protein. It is one of the secrets to controlling your appetite and losing weight. If you want to save time, cook up about a pound of lean ground beef. Use some of it right away—for quick tacos or sloppy joes, for example—then refrigerate the rest to utilize in other meals over the next few days.

The Supermarket Deli to the Rescue

Of course, we don't always have time to prepare a home-cooked meal. Happily, there is an easy solution. These days people stop at the supermarket on their way home not to buy ingredients for dinner, but for already prepared deli meals that only need to be heated up or scooped straight from the container onto the plate. They're called "prepared meals," and more and more supermarkets are turning over large swaths of floor space to them.

A 2004 survey by the Food Marketing Institute found that 27 percent of respondents said they got most of their take-out meals from supermarkets, compared with 35 percent from fast-food restaurants and 18 percent from full-service eateries. That's nearly twice as many as in 2002. Meanwhile, industry researchers predict that dinners from the take-out counter or grocery freezer will likely overtake homemade meals within the next five years.

Most grocery stores offer the basics, such as fried and rotisserie chickens, salad bars, and so on. If you're lucky enough to live near an upscale grocery such as Whole Foods or Wegman's, you know that today's takeout can border on the exotic. These chains offer hot buffet lines, sushi, salad and soup bars, and even foreign cuisines—not to mention pizza, chicken wings, hoagies, and other delectable treats.

And choices are likely to increase even further since at Whole Foods, for example, these ready-to-go meals already represent about 10 percent of the store's sales. Convenience stores are also getting in on the act. Just about every "quick-stop" store has added hot food stations and deli lines.

Despite the wholesome image projected by many of the upscale groceries, their ready-to-go meals are just as likely as those from the corner fast-food joint to contain excess fat, calories, and salt. But some of these entrées and side dishes are lean and nutritious enough to fit perfectly into any weight-loss plan, though it's not always easy to tell which one. Some supermarkets post nutritional information in the display cases or on their Web sites, but the majority do not. After reading this far, you should have a good idea how to make the best choices.

Rotisserie chickens are a case in point. All you have to do is look at the glistening, golden-brown skin to know that it's going to drop some fat into your diet. Actually, one serving of bird will probably have less than 300 calories and about 4 grams of saturated fat. That's not bad if you're including it with other foods—not so great if that's all you're eating and you pick the carcass clean. Nonetheless, these chickens contain a hefty helping of salt, so watch out if you have high blood pressure.

How about that ready-to-go seafood salad? If it's made with olive oil, go for it. If, on the other hand, it's a creamy salad with whopping amounts of mayo, you'll wind up getting as many calories as you would with a cheeseburger and soft drink.

Ready-to-go meals have one great advantage: You can control exactly what you get—the main meal, the sides, the salad, and everything else. If you shop with weight loss in mind, you can come home with the perfect blend of lean protein, low-glycemic carbs, and healthy fats in less time than it takes for a restaurant meal and almost as fast as pulling through a fast-food drive-up lane.

Given all the choices from the deli cases, salad bars, and full-service bakeries, you're left with the crucial one to either stick to your calorie budget or blow it big-time. Here are a few ways to enjoy the convenience of ready-to-go foods as part of a smart-eating plan.

Mix prepared and fresh   Sure, you can buy a complete meal at the grocery store, but that can add up to big bucks and even more total calories. Better to take the middle ground. Buy an entrée that you really like, especially one that you wouldn't normally make at home. Once it's in the cart, pick up some broccoli or baby carrots in the produce department. Or grab a can of string beans. At home, you can quickly cook some rice and steam the vegetables before warming your entrée. You'll cut your cooking time to almost nothing, while enjoying a dinner that's almost customized for calorie control.

Don't forget the salad bar   Load a box with mixed greens, tomatoes, onions, olives, or anything else you like. You'll bump up your vegetable servings for the day with hardly any calories, assuming that you don't add all those toppings and creamy dressing.

Watch for hidden fats   Prepared foods and frozen heat-and-eat dinners that are labeled with nutritional information make it easy to monitor your calorie and fat intake. In the absence of such labels, all you can do is look for clues. Pools of oil at the bottom of containers are a pretty good tip-off. Creamy sauces and dressings are invariably loaded with fat. If nothing else, ask the person behind the counter how the foods were prepared.

Don't order by the pound   Most prepared foods are sold by weight rather than size. Resist taking home more than you really need. An easy way to control portion sizes is to ask for just enough to feed a certain number of people. Just remember, it's in the store's interest to give you more, not less.

Ladle some ready-to-go soup   Most soups are low in fat, unless they are cream-based. You can cut back the fat and calories even further by getting a vegetable or bean soup rather than a meat one. Remember, starting a meal with soup is optimal for weight loss because you'll eat less of the richer, higher-calorie foods and consume fewer calories overall.

Beware of Chinese take-out   A lot of supermarkets now include impressive lineups of ready-to-eat Chinese meals, such as sesame noodles, twice-cooked pork, and those hard-to-resist chicken wings. Buy these at your own peril. A lot of these dishes are fried; those that aren't are usually drenched in oil. You'll get at least as much fat and calories in this section as you would at your neighborhood Chinese restaurant.

Plan for leftovers   Prepared foods are natural time-savers, so why not double your savings and cut back on calories by "stretching" the main dish? If you're buying a rotisserie chicken, serve parts of it with a salad and vegetables for one meal and use the leftovers in a stir-fry or Caesar salad the next day.

Ready-to-Go Entrées

The larger supermarket chains offer dozens of main-dish, heat-and-serve meals, from sole stuffed with lobster and shrimp to pork rolls filled with spinach and cheese. Take them home and pop them in a 350-degree oven, watch the news for twenty or thirty minutes, and your food will be ready to eat. It doesn't get easier than that—unless you buy an entrée that's already hot and steaming. And many of these foods are far more elaborate than anything we usually make at home.

Entrées typically supply the lion's share of fat and calories, but that has more to do with the way most people eat than the actual calories in the foods themselves. Sliced beef marinated in a rich wine sauce will probably have more saturated fat and calories than a whole-grain or potato side dish. It's not a problem if you set aside about a quarter of your plate for the entrée and fill up the rest with low-calorie side dishes. This balance is ideal for weight loss and long-term health.

Seafood

If everyone would substitute seafood for just one or two red-meat servings a week, we'd have much less heart disease and other health problems. Bottom line: If you want to lose weight and live longer, eat healthy fish at least twice a week.

Of course, even the healthiest, leanest foods undergo startling transformations when they're drenched in butter, covered in breading, and plunged into hot oil or grease. Fish is no exception. When you're shopping for ready-to-go seafood at the supermarket, look for fish that has been steamed, poached, or broiled rather than fried, with minimum butter added. Here are a few examples.

Try pan-seared salmon Most supermarkets offer one or more variations of pan-cooked fish. Thanks to the high heat of the cooking oil, little is absorbed. A serving of pan-seared wild salmon only has about 250 calories and 1.5 grams of saturated fat. The total fat may look high (typically around 10 or 12 grams), but since most of that is the healthy type, it's definitely a good-for-you entrée.

Celebrate with crab cakes Even people who don't like seafood usually love crab cakes. They're higher in calories than most fish (about 400 in a 6-ounce serving) and have a little more saturated fat, but they're still lean enough to eat without guilt. Just don't drench them in butter or tartar sauce. Fresh-squeezed lemon juice with chopped parsley or cilantro is your best low-calorie choice.

Roll with sushi Few foods are better when you're trying to lose weight. Most sushi rolls, made of seaweed wrapped around rice (or rice molded around seaweed) with a little bit of cooked or raw fish, have only about 150 calories. They don't look like much, but because of the rice they can fill you up faster than you might think.

Steamed snapper with vegetables   Steaming fish is about the best way to cook it. Steaming adds no calories or saturated fat. Combining the snapper with sautéed vegetables and small amounts of olive oil and garlic yields a very healthy weight-loss meal. You're looking at about 330 calories and usually less than 4 grams saturated fat.

Watch out for "crusted" fish   Most supermarkets offer one or more varieties of fish crusted with breading or nuts. As soon as any kind of coating is thrown into the mix, the calories and fat shoot upward. A serving of pecan-crusted tilapia, for example, can harbor more than 600 calories and 30 grams of fat. That's not a diet killer by any stretch, but the amount of fat is borderline in a healthy diet.

Chicken and Meat Dishes

More than a few studies have suggested that a vegetarian diet—no meat, no milk, and no eggs—is nearly ideal for lowering cholesterol, preventing heart disease and stroke, and losing weight. A recent study at George Washington University found that women who followed a low-fat vegetarian diet for fourteen weeks lost an average of 13 pounds, compared to the 8-pound average loss by women who adhered to a standard low-fat diet.

Yet that's not how most Americans eat, nor is it really necessary. There's nothing wrong with including meat in your diet, even red meats such as beef and lamb. Admittedly, they are often higher in calories than plant foods. But it's fine to enjoy a meat entrée a few times a week or to use smaller amounts of meat in soups, stews, and stir-fries. No matter how you slice it, a 16-ounce porterhouse isn't going to do your arteries or your hips any good if you eat one every day. But some meat-based prepared meals from the supermarket can give you the best of both worlds: the rich, satisfying flavor of meat with relatively few calories and little saturated fat. Here are a few examples.

Roasted chicken   You can pick up these ready-to-go birds at just about any supermarket. They're always a reasonable choice. You're looking at about 130 calories and 8 grams of fat per serving, with only about 3 grams coming from satu-rated fat. As long as you limit your serving size to 3 or 4 ounces and fill the rest of your plate with whole grains, beans, or vegetables, you could eat like this most nights and still stay in a weight-loss zone. If you're really serious about watching your weight and lowering your cholesterol, peel off the skin. A whole roasted chicken will lose about 51 grams of fat and 567 calories when you do. My only warn-ing is the added salt. Remember, if you have high blood pressure, you may want to pass on this.

Chicken with fennel and leeks   I came across this hot entrée at Wegman's. Talk about an elegant feast! It's obviously not as lean as a plain, roasted chicken, but with 490 calories and 3.5 grams of saturated fat per serving, it's a heck of a lot healthier than a restaurant meal—and faster than anything you can make at home.

Roast pork   You probably remember the advertising cam-paign that referred to pork as the "other white meat." It's not quite true that pork is as lean as chicken, but it's leaner than beef. A ready-to-go roast pork dish from the supermarket "heat and serve line" will probably have about 250 calories and 12 grams fat. Compare that to a grilled New York strip with about 761 calories and 56 grams of fat.

Meat lasagna   I wouldn't call this a low-calorie food. I include it here to show you how easy it is to go wrong in the prepared food aisle. A dish like this probably contains about 600 calories, which still isn't bad compared to something similar at a restaurant. But with 19 grams of saturated fat, it's not the kind of meal you'd want to eat very often if you're trying to control your weight and health. On the other hand, if you just got the macaroni and cheese, without meat, you'd save about 480 calories.

Sandwiches   The deli departments in some of today's supermarkets are truly outstanding. You can find dozens of varieties of sliced meats and cheeses and a wide selection of breads and rolls. If possible, always order your sandwich on whole-grain bread or rolls. Load them up with vegetable toppings and pass on the mayo and other "special sauces." Also remember to keep your meats lean. Roast beef is a better choice than salami, chicken is better than proscuitto and cheese, and turkey breast is always a good call.

Fried foods   Anything that's fried is going to jack up the calorie count higher than you would imagine. A Cajun-fried chicken sandwich, for example, will set you back about 520 calories and 24 grams of fat, even more than a chicken BLT (410 calories, 11 grams of fat). Try to minimize or completely avoid foods like these.

Side Dishes

Hooray for sides! Even a small supermarket might have a few dozen choices—and the big chains, such as Wild Oats or Albertsons, might have close to a hundred. We Americans have the unfortunate tendency to think of side dishes as "extras"—something to complement the main dish, which is usually meat or fish. Ideally, for weight loss as well as good health in general, it should be the other way around. We'd all be better off if we made whole grains, vegetables, beans, and salads the stars of any meal, with meat in a supporting role.

Supermarket side dishes can be one of the main sources of hidden fat and calories. In the absence of clear nutritional information, your best bet is to avoid anything conspicuously creamy or oily. Plain and simple work best when you want to slim down. For example:

Vegetables and beans   Most supermarkets sell several variations of bean and vegetable dishes and marinated salads. They're almost always a good choice, although the marinades can be surprisingly high in fat. A red bean and corn salad, for example, probably has in the neighborhood of 240 calories and 13 grams of total fat. That's not terrible, but you wouldn't want to have a triple serving.

Fruit salads   I've seen enticing combinations of grapes, nuts, cheese, pears, and other fruits and seeds. A pear and cheese salad will come in at about 200 calories and maybe 5 grams of total fat. Good choice!

Marinated mushrooms   This is another supermarket standard. Once again, the oil in the marinade is going to bump up the fat—but hardly to alarming proportions. Ask to see if the oil used is olive oil. If it is, go for it. Count on about 160 calories and 14 grams of fat.

Roasted vegetables   Just about any vegetable can be roasted, which caramelizes the sugars and gives a sweet, slightly smoky flavor. Roasted vegetables are a good choice for managing calories. A serving will usually have about 120 calories and less than 2 grams of fat.

Whole-grain salads   These can be quite yummy. I love curried couscous, Mediterranean orzo with wheat berries, and seven-grain salads. As with the other side dishes, however, some can be a little high in calories and fat. The multigrain salad clocks in at 240 calories. Not bad, but not great, either. Tabbouleh, a Mediterranean grain dish loaded with nutritious parsley, is a better choice with only 140 calories per serving.

At the Salad Bar

I wish I'd grown up with the amazing salad bars now found in just about every supermarket. The selection of greens is often as good as what you'll find in the produce aisles. Plus they include plenty of extras: olives, pasta salads, fruit salads, artichoke hearts, and more. If you like raw onions, don't skimp on them! They're packed with a nutrient called *quercetin* (also found in red wine), which is a definite heart savior that also bolsters your immune system. Many of my patients tell me that eating lots of onions seemed to increase their weight loss. Give it a try.

There are far too many kinds of prepared salads for me to cover them all. Here are some of the more popular ones and how they rate for health and weight loss.

Pasta salads   These can vary widely in calorie content. Definitely choose salads that are dressed in some type of olive oil-herb mix. You'll still get some fat calories, but the fat will be almost entirely the healthy, monounsaturated kind. Creamy dressings are another story. I noticed one broccoli and ziti salad, for example, with about 330 calories and 27 grams of fat. That's too much when you're trying to watch your weight.

Potato salads   They tend to be too high in fat. Most stores offer a variety of lower-fat options, such as potatoes in Dijon mustard or balsamic vinegar dressing, instead of mayonnaise. With these, you'll probably get under 150 calories and less than 7 or 8 grams of fat. That's reasonable.

Slaw and Asian salads   These are among the leaner salads, marinated in oil and vinegar rather than drenched in mayo. A basic coleslaw without mayo contains about 90 calories, with 4 grams of fat. An Asian cabbage salad runs in the same fat-and-calorie range, but with a bit more of a vinegary taste.

Seafood salads   Most tend to be on the creamy side, although the benefits of the omega-3s from the fish can offset a few extra calories. Expect to get about 180 calories and 14 grams of fat (very little of which is saturated).

Great Finds in the Freezer

Today's frozen meals have little in common with the high-fat, high-salt, and high-sugar TV dinners of yesteryear. It's relatively easy to find products that are low in fat and calories, while providing a good balance of protein, fat, and carbohydrates. None of that matters, of course, if they taste like the boxes they come in. Here are some of my favorite choices for weight control as well as taste.

Ethnic Gourmet Bowl Pad Thai with Tofu   This comes with rice noodles in peanut sauce, along with a mix of vegetables and tofu. With a combination like that, you don't need to add anything else. Contains: *460 calories and 8 grams fat.*

Lean Cuisine Baked Fish with Cheddar Shells   It's a convenient way to get one of your weekly fish servings, although the fish (Alaskan pollock) isn't as high in omega-3s as salmon or mackerel. Serve this with a whole grain, a steamed vegetable, and a salad to round out the meal. Contains: *310 calories and 8 grams fat.*

Michelina's Lean Gourmet Roasted Sirloin Supreme   Not quite a meal by itself, but if you throw in a few sides, such as a baked potato and a fresh green salad, it's filling enough for any appetite and will help you lose weight at the same time. Contains: *230 calories and 5 grams fat.*

Healthy Choice Chicken Breast and Vegetables   The protein-to-carb ratio in this is nearly perfect for weight control, and it's tasty enough to feel like a dinner treat. Thumbs up! Contains: *230 calories and 5 grams fat.*

Linda McCartney Spicy Thai Veggie Pizza   The crust is almost as good as one you'd get from a real pizza oven; and the mix of grilled vegetables, mozzarella, and Thai peanut sauce is surprisingly delicious. Contains: *320 calories and 9 grams fat.*

Hot Tips for Cutting the Fat

If you've been on any kind of diet in the last few years (and who hasn't?), you may have heard that you should get rid of all the fat in your diet. That's old school. Hardly any respected expert endorses this approach anymore. True, it *is* healthy to cut back on saturated fats, but there are the "good" fats that you can—and should—eat more of. And food that's been stripped of fat has all the flavor and mouth-appeal of cardboard. While there are two main ways to reduce (not eliminate) fat from the diet, only one gets talked about very much.

Most fat-reducing advice focuses on ingredients: Get rid of butter, use spray instead of cooking oil, buy "low-fat" everything. It's good advice, but it's only half of the equation. *How* you cook has just as much impact on the fat in your diet as *what* you cook with. For example, if you like frying foods, you can pretty much abandon hope of losing pounds. That's because cooking oils and other fats add a lot of extra calories to an otherwise low-cal piece of fish or chicken. Here are some smarter cooking methods that bring out the flavor of foods, preserve their nutrients, and minimize your intake of unnecessary fat.

Baking Very few baked foods, apart from desserts, require any added fat whatsoever. With covered casseroles, oven-baked stews, or baked potatoes, the foods' own juices will keep them moist and tender during cooking. Roasting does the same thing, except you use higher temperatures.

Grilling Whether you're using charcoal briquettes or propane, get your barbie really *hot*. Exposing thin strips of meats or vegetables to direct heat sears the surface of the food, trapping the natural juices inside. No need for added fat, though when grilling fish, you might want to brush some oil on the grate to keep it from sticking. Broiling in the oven has the same effect as grilling, except that the heat comes from the top rather than the bottom.

Poaching Simmering ingredients in water or flavored liquids, such as chicken stock, is probably the best way to achieve a fork-tender texture. Always cover the pot to trap steam and speed cooking time.

Sautéing Like frying, this requires adding oil to the pan. But unlike frying, you only use a scant amount. When you cut the ingredients into thin, small pieces, all of the surface areas quickly come into contact with the hot oil for uniform cooking. Stir-frying is essentially the same technique,

Calorie-Shaving Substitutes

When you look at the ingredients in most traditional recipes—gobs of butter, tablespoons of sugar, and enough eggs to start your own chicken farm—it's hard to imagine that their authors have ever worn anything smaller than a size fourteen.

Don't be afraid to tinker with recipes. Even if you're more interested in playing with taste than knocking down calories, you can almost always substitute healthier ingredients without sacrificing taste or texture. Here are some tips:

Recipe calls for	Substitute
Bacon	Turkey bacon, Canadian bacon, or lean prosciutto
Butter	Applesauce for half the butter called for
Eggs	Two egg whites instead of one whole one
Enriched pasta	Whole-wheat pasta
Meat	Chopped mushrooms, whole grains
White rice	Brown rice, wild rice, or quinoa
Salad dressing	Fat-free dressing or herbal vinaigrettes
Salt	Salt-free spice or herb blends
Sugar	Cinnamon, allspice, or vanilla for half the sugar called for

except you usually use a larger pan, such as a wok, and stir frequently to prevent sticking and uneven cooking.

Steaming   This is one of the simplest cooking techniques, as well as the fastest and most healthful. Food suspended in a basket above simmering water or stock or placed in a double boiler can absorb water and stay tender without any need for added fat.

Five Kitchen Gadgets You Can't Live Without

Why do most people abandon their weight-loss efforts? The two main reasons they give are a lack of time and higher food costs, though I'm not sure I really believe either one. But let's assume they're being honest. With the right kitchen gear, anyone can knock both of these obstacles squarely off the path to good health and proper weight. In fact, some pieces of kitchen equipment work so efficiently that prep time becomes a nonfactor. Most of these gadgets easily pay for themselves because you'll waste less food and won't want to dine out as often. They help you cook faster and eat better at home. So what are these miracle machines?

Blender   Better yet, a mini-blender with a one- to three-cup capacity. These small blenders clean up faster than full-sized models and are actually more versatile, good for grinding flaxseed (for the heart-healthy omega-3s), blending fruits and liquids into smoothies, and making your own low-fat salad dressings and sauces. Those sauces can range from a basic pesto to fiery-hot chili concoctions. If you check out the prices of these condiments on your next shopping trip, you'll be amazed how much you can save by making them yourself.

Kitchen scissors   No kidding, they really make a difference. For example, if you're using more fresh herbs in order to cut back on salt, scissors are perfect for snipping them quickly into tiny, recipe-ready bits. It's much faster than dicing with a knife. You can also use them to snip fish and poultry into small pieces for low-fat cooking, or trim excess fat from beef, pork, or poultry. Joyce Chen makes an excellent pair of all-purpose kitchen scissors.

Rice cooker   Once you see the wisdom in cutting back on processed foods, you will begin replacing them with rice and whole grains. You can cook brown and white rice in a stove-top pot, but it's tricky to get it right. That's why I have an automatic rice cooker. It turns off when the rice is perfectly done. You're free to attend to other things.

Skimmer   When making soups or stews, you'll see globs of fat rising to the surface. Get rid of them, because they're just extra pounds waiting to camp out on your body. A skimmer strips the fat off the surface of liquid, making your soups and stews lighter and healthier.

Steamer   Like using the microwave, cooking with steam prepares food quickly with no oil added. It also preserves the color, flavor, and nutrients that are lost when you boil. To steam vegetables (or fish or anything else), first bring the water to a boil. Layer the ingredients on the steamer, and cover. Be sure the hot water won't touch the food, because it will leach away nutrients and destroy the taste and texture.

Ten Healthy Dishes You Can Make in a Flash

Eating out is fun. I love it as much as anyone. But eating in is fun, too, especially when you can knock out delicious, super-fast, and super-nutritious meals that contain just a few hundred calories per serving. A few such home-cooked meals every week will keep your health and weight on track, even if you've been ordering at the fast food drive-thru windows. Here are ten super-fast, super-healthful, super-slimming dishes you can whip up in minutes. (For more low-cal, quick recipes, go to our free Web site at www.thefastfooddiet.com.) Eating these meals a few times throughout the week will help you shed a pound or two a week without having to make any other changes.

Steamed Fish with Pesto   In the mood for something elegant and light? Nothing's easier than steamed fish and vegetables topped with a little pesto sauce.

1. Combine in a blender a cup of fresh basil leaves, a tablespoon of pine nuts, a fresh tomato, and a clove of fresh garlic. Add one to two tablespoons of olive oil, and blend until smooth.

2. Put a steamer basket in a saucepan. Add water to about half an inch below the bottom of the steamer basket. Bring the water to a boil, put a filet of salmon or sole in the steamer. Cover and steam until tender, usually about five minutes.

3. While the fish is steaming, chop some broccoli, baby bok choy, or another vegetable of your choice. Put in a microwave-safe dish, cover, and microwave until tender.

4. Spoon the pesto over the fish and vegetables, and serve. If this meal seems a little light, you can add a cup of steamed brown rice or a few slices of fresh whole-grain bread. Pesto goes with everything.

Five-Minute Marinara   This Italian classic is traditionally used as a topping for pasta, but it's equally good on baked potatoes, skinless chicken breasts, toasted sourdough bread (to make bruschetta), or brown rice.

1. Coarsely chop one large onion, two large tomatoes, and two cloves of garlic. Heat a little olive oil in a medium-size saucepan. Sauté the onion until it's almost tender, then add the garlic. When the garlic is just lightly brown, add the tomato, along with a splash of balsamic vinegar,

a few capers, and salt and pepper to taste (easy on the salt). You can also add anchovies and sliced green olives.

2. Reduce the heat to simmer and cook five minutes, stirring occasionally.

Grilled Mediterranean Vegetables   Cooking vegetables on the grill gives them a sweet, smoky flavor—and you don't have to heat up the kitchen during the warm months. This dish is a perfect companion to roast chicken, pasta, or steamed fish. It's also hearty enough for a main course if you add some garlic bread and a crisp green salad.

1. Chop or slice three or four of your favorite vegetables so that they're all about the same size: a few large red onions, Italian frying or bell peppers, eggplant, summer squash, and asparagus make a good mix.

2. Put the vegetables in a bowl, and add one to two tablespoons of olive oil. Toss well, transfer to a grill basket, and place on the hot grill. Shake the basket vigorously at least once a minute or, if the vegetables are held tightly by the basket, turn it over. Grill for five to ten minutes, or until all the vegetables are tender, but not wilted.

3. Transfer to a bowl, stir in red wine or balsamic vinegar to taste, and serve.

Cinnamon French Toast   This family favorite is a snap to make—and if you replace the whole eggs with egg whites, you can knock down the fat to almost nothing.

1. In a large bowl or rectangular baking dish, combine half a cup of skim milk, half a cup of egg whites, ¼ teaspoon of vanilla, and ¼ teaspoon of cinnamon.

2. One at a time, add thick slices of sourdough, oat bran, or whole wheat bread to the milk-egg mix. Turn the pieces to thoroughly coat both sides.

3. Coat a large, no-stick frying pan with nonstick spray. Place over medium heat until hot. Transfer the bread slices to the pan, and brown both sides evenly. Then top with maple syrup or jam.

Chicken Curry in a Hurry   Who says you can't impress guests without spending hours in the kitchen? This rich, exotic curry dish takes almost no time to prepare and is filling enough—and low enough in calories—that you can eat it as often as you like.

1. In a small bowl, combine ½ cup yogurt, a few tablespoons of nonfat mayonnaise, ¼ cup finely chopped onions, 1 teaspoon of freshly grated ginger root, and 2 teaspoons of curry powder.

2. Cut two chicken breasts into half-inch strips. Coat with ground black pepper and a sprinkling of ground cumin or paprika.

3. Drizzle a little olive oil into a nonstick pan and place it on medium heat. When the pan is hot, add the chicken, turning frequently until all sides are brown. Combine the chicken with the yogurt-curry mixture and stir well.

4. Serve over brown rice or whole-grain noodles.

Tomato-Simmered Salmon   This dish is so quickly prepared that it could serve as a fast lunch, yet it also makes an elegant supper. And you probably have most of the ingredients already.

1. Coarsely chop two large tomatoes. Dice a few tablespoons each of onion, carrot, and celery.

2. Drizzle a little olive oil into a nonstick skillet and place it on medium heat. When the pan is hot, quickly sear one or more salmon fillets. Cook no more than thirty seconds per side, then set aside on a plate.

3. Add the onion, carrot, and celery to the fish pan, stirring frequently to pick up the juices. Sauté until soft, then add the tomatoes and a splash of balsamic vinegar. Stir well, then layer the fish on top. Cover, cook about three minutes on low heat, turn the fish, and cook three more minutes on the other side.

4. Serve on a bed of brown rice.

Vegetarian Stir-Fry   You won't necessarily lose weight on a vegetarian diet, but it's pretty hard not to, because a plant-based diet naturally provides an abundance of bulky fiber and insulin-regulating complex carbs along with its antioxidant-rich fruits and vegetables. Just don't slather on the oil! That will add back a lot of the calories you dodge by cutting out (or cutting back on) meat.

1. Chop one yellow onion and one bell pepper in large pieces. Dice two carrots, and mince two cloves of garlic. Slice about half a cup of mushrooms.

2. Drip a little olive oil in a wok and heat over a high flame. Add one teaspoon of black bean sauce. Stir constantly for about thirty seconds, then lower the heat to medium. Add the vegetables and continuing stirring until they're soft. Then add the mushrooms and, if you have them, some bean sprouts.

3. Sprinkle in some low-sodium soy sauce, and serve over rice.

4. If you're not a vegetarian, you can add about half a pound of flank steak to the recipe. Cut the meat into thin strips, marinate in low-sodium soy sauce for half an hour, and cook in the wok before you add the vegetables.

Fast Frittata   The next time you have friends over for a weekend brunch, whip up this robust, delicious omelet for them.

1. Whisk four eggs in a bowl. Season with salt and pepper, and add a quick splash of low-fat or nonfat milk.

2. Heat a skillet over medium heat. Drizzle in olive oil, and maybe one teaspoon of butter for flavor. When the oil is hot, sauté ¼ cup chopped onion, one bunch chopped green onions, and one diced tomato for about three minutes, then add the eggs.

3. When the top of the mixture starts to cook well, add ½ sliced avocado and ¼ cup grated low-fat cheddar cheese. Turn off the heat, and leave the frittata in the pan until the cheese starts to melt. Lift pieces out with a spatula and serve.

Quick Blueberry-Peach Crumble   This is probably the easiest pie recipe you'll ever make. Mmm—delicious!

1. Peel and cut four peaches into slices. Add to a bowl with one pint of blueberries. Add the juice of half a lemon, a sprinkle of cinnamon, and ⅛ cup brown sugar.

2. In another bowl, combine ½ cup flour, ½ cup one-minute rolled oats, two heaping tablespoons of brown sugar, ¼ cup applesauce, and ¼ cup butter. Mix with your hands until the ingredients are blended to a crumbly texture.

3. Add the fruit to a glass pie plate and cover with the flour mixture. Bake in a 350-degree oven for forty minutes. Let cool for half an hour, then serve.

Yummy Lemon-Ginger Chicken   Low-fat and weight-loss cookbooks always have a zillion recipes for chicken breasts. But how much chicken can you really stand? Well, with this recipe you will want to eat some more.

1. Cube two chicken breasts, and sauté in a skillet with a little olive oil, using medium-high heat. When the chicken is almost done, remove from the skillet and set aside.

Add two teaspoons of freshly grated ginger and two cloves of minced garlic to the skillet and return it to the fire. Let brown, then squeeze in the juice of one lemon. Add one teaspoon brown sugar and stir well. Bring to a simmer and continue cooking.

2. Dissolve one teaspoon of cornstarch in a little warm water, stirring well so it doesn't clump. Stir into the lemon-ginger mix in the skillet, then add back the chicken. Cook for one additional minute.

3. Serve over brown rice or noodles.

(If you'd like additional quick, nutritious, weight-loss recipes like these, you can find them on our free Web site at www.thefastfooddiet.com.)

CHAPTER 9

The Fast-Food Diet for Kids

A dults aren't the only ones with weight problems. The number of children in North America who are overweight has doubled in the last few decades. One in five children is now overweight. One in three children born in the United States within the past five years is projected to develop diabetes in his or her life. For Latino children, the figure is one out of two.

Obesity and overweight are such serious problems that public health professionals warn that our children may be the first generation who won't live longer than their parents! But with so much fast-food advertising targeting them, how do you rear kids who don't constantly crave junk food and turn up their noses to real food?

It's not easy. Children are bombarded with even more food advertisements than adults are. According to Kelly D. Brownell, Ph.D., one of the country's top obesity researchers,

151

the average American child sees ten thousand food advertisements a year—and that's just on television. Most of these ads are for fast foods, super-sweet cereals, soft drinks, and candy. A study of children ages six through eight found that 70 percent of them believed that fast food was healthier than the foods they ate at home.

Fast-food and restaurant chains take every opportunity to polish their "kid-friendly" images, offering menu items such as Happy Meals and linking popular cartoon characters to particular food products. The chains know very well that lifelong food preferences start early. They're right on. Nearly half of parents with six- to eleven-year-olds eat out at least once a week, and about 20 percent do it more often. The consumption of fast food by our children has increased five times since 1970. Every day, nearly a third of all American children eat fast food, which adds an extra *six pounds* to the average kid's weight per year.

Once again, nature is partly to blame. Children have a natural preference for sweet and fatty foods, such as ice cream. They're genetically programmed to initially dislike more bitter foods—which includes, unfortunately, healthy items such as spinach and broccoli. Children must taste a new food up to ten times before it starts to taste familiar and good to them. Rather than deal with whiny, unhappy children, many parents understandably give in and let their kids order whatever they want from the menu.

Is there a way to short-circuit restaurant food fights and, at the same time, help children establish healthier eating habits? Yes, but given the offerings at most restaurant chains, it's a challenge. Here are a few tips for keeping those junk-food calories to a minimum, while starting your kids off on a path to lifelong healthy diet habits.

Don't trust the "kids' menu"   When you add up all of the saturated fat, trans fat, sugar, and calories in the foods offered specifically to our children, it's easy to see why they are heavier than any kids in human history—and why they face a much higher risk of diabetes and heart disease later in life. Virtually every chain includes fried chicken on the children's menu, plus hamburgers and cheeseburgers, macaroni and cheese, corn dogs or hot dogs, and cheesy pizza. And of course, everything comes with french fries and a complimentary soft drink. Talk about calorie overload! The only real advantage to children's menus is that they offer smaller portions. My advice is, when you can't find anything that's truly healthy, order from the adult menu and ask for a reduced portion. Or take home what's left.

Mix things up   Even when kids' menus do offer a few healthy entrées, they hardly ever provide nutritious side dishes. So mix things up. At Cracker Barrel, for example, the kids' menu offers Grilled Chicken Tenderloin with only 110 calories and 1 gram of saturated fat. That's a great choice, especially if you pair it with some baby carrots or green beans from the adult side of the menu. Another good idea is to swap out the soft drink for a glass of milk or orange juice. With a meal like that, you're looking at roughly 320 calories, which isn't bad at all.

Order quickly   Even a ten-minute wait at a sit-down restaurant is too long for squirmy children. They typically entertain themselves by polishing off the breadsticks, white bread, or other carbohydrates that are waiting on the table. These foods almost guarantee weight gain and extra sugar cravings later. Then they're full. So as soon as you sit down, ask the waiter to bring a fruit cup, which is a lot healthier than the bread. Or ask that your child's food be served right away.

Cut down the portions   The average child age four to eight needs only about 1,500 calories a day. Yet most restaurants dish up enough food for kids with the biggest appetites— namely, twelve-year-old boys. You can easily wind up with a meal that supplies 700 calories or more. That's way too much for young children. Yet once the food is in front of them, many boys and girls will clean their plate, even if they aren't that hungry. Especially if they see Mom and Dad doing the same. Remember, you can always split a kid's meal between two children, or set half aside and take it home in a doggy bag.

Dodge the burgers   By the time you add the fries and a soft drink to a hamburger, you're looking at a meal approaching 1,000 calories. You'll do better with spaghetti or macaroni, which usually appear on most children's menus. As long as you throw in a vegetable side (from the adult part of the menu, if necessary), you can keep the calories between 300 and 400, with relatively little fat.

Skip the ice cream   Most children's menus include ice cream or a sundae. It's often part of the meal, which seems like a bargain—until you realize that a sundae topped with choco-late sauce and whipped cream can add more than 700 calo-ries. Some kids' menus offer fruit for dessert. I suggest you order it. Or, to preserve family harmony, you can always whisper to the waiter not to mention dessert. If your child balks, put your foot down. No matter how much kids may protest, this will be a lot less unpleasant for them than daily insulin shots if they develop diabetes.

Shop around   Quite a few of the chains, possibly worried about future lawsuits, have started offering healthier children's meals. There aren't a lot of choices right now, but at least the trend is starting. Here are some examples

(for others check out our free Web site at www
.thefastfooddiet.com).

- Some McDonald's and Wendy's offer kids' meals that substitute milk (or juice) for soda, and fruit for fries.

- Legal Sea Foods serves a fruit and vegetable with every entrée for kids.

- Red Lobster's children's menu now includes grilled fish, grilled chicken, and snow crab legs—much healthier than the fried fish that used to dominate the menu. But refuse the little pot of liquid butter that comes along, or tell the waiter to skip it beforehand.

- The Old Spaghetti Factory includes a salad or apple-sauce with all children's meals, along with a choice of milk or apple juice.

- Chili's kids' menu used to emphasize "fried." It now offers a grilled chicken sandwich or platter, pasta with healthy tomato sauce, and a choice of healthier side dishes.

CHAPTER 10

The Fast-Food Diet Vitamins and Supplements

P eople who eat fast food regularly need extra vitamins and nutrients—more so than the average person. And I'll tell you why . . .

One reason is that the majority of fast foods are deficient in important vitamins, minerals, and other vital nutrients such as fiber. Moreover, fast foods contain substances that can increase free radical damage to your cells and tissues, while also causing widespread inflammation. Both will make you look and feel older and have been associated with increased risk of heart disease, Alzheimer's, and various types of cancers.

Another, perhaps more important, reason is that many fast foods contain potentially harmful substances such as saturated fat, sugar, and inflammatory agents that can be neutralized by certain vitamins and supplements so health problems are less likely to develop. This chapter will explain the specifics so you can be sure you are safeguarding your health.

A century ago, deficiency diseases due to a lack of vitamins and minerals were among the leading causes of poor health. Doctors understood that a nutritious diet is important, but they didn't know just how important until the science of nutrition developed and proved it.

These days, the old-fashioned types of dietary deficiencies aren't all that common in North America. People in other parts of the world aren't as lucky. Here food is abundant and relatively affordable. Even if you never paid the slightest attention to nutrition, you'd probably get most of the minimal amounts of vitamins and minerals just by eating regular meals.

Doctors have identified certain core nutrients, along with the minimal amounts people need to prevent yesteryear's deficiency diseases—such as rickets (from a lack of vitamin D), scurvy (not enough vitamin C), and pellagra (low niacin). *But that's not enough to stay truly healthy.* Optimal health requires optimal nutrition. Unfortunately, fast food and many one-per-day multiple vitamins don't provide that. While many popular brands may promise to be complete "A to Z" products, most of them merely provide cosmetic traces of essential nutrients. I routinely tell my patients to carefully read the nutrition facts on each product label and not to purchase an item simply because it is advertised as the kitchen sink of nutrients.

Take folate, also known as folic acid, for example. The recommended daily amount of this B vitamin is 200 micrograms (mcg.). This is the minimal dose necessary to prevent spina bifida, a terrible birth defect that often occurs in the newborns of young mothers who eat fast food regularly. But this amount is insufficient to guard against other health problems.

Studies published in the *Journal of the American Medical Association* and the *American Journal of Clinical Nutrition* have shown a significant heart-protective benefit from taking at least 400 to 800 mcg. of folic acid daily. Researchers also report that higher levels of folate block certain cancers by protecting your DNA from damage. In fact, about half of all cancers caused by DNA damage are due to insufficient folate. This has been proven by solid medical research, yet many doctors still hesitate to recommend vitamins and other supplements that contain folate levels above the minimal standards.

One thing is certain: It's almost impossible to reap the cancer-preventing benefits of folate if you eat a lot of fast food—and don't make up the difference with nutritious meals at home or by taking a vitamin containing at least 600 to 800 mcg. of folate daily. If everyone would take this one simple action, the risk of breast cancer would drop 25 to 50 percent, and the risk of colon cancer would drop anywhere from 25 to 69 percent. You can't buy a cheaper cancer "insurance policy."

Here's another example. The average person needs only about fifteen minutes of sun exposure a day to get adequate amounts of vitamin D. (It's synthesized in the body in response to ultraviolet light.) But guess what? The vast majority of North Americans, as many as 87 percent, don't receive sufficient vitamin D because they either don't go outside enough or aren't getting it in their diet or from a vitamin pill. This lack of vitamin D almost guarantees weak bones (osteoporosis) and increases the risk of cancer, especially of the prostate and the breast.

I believe many doctors and health professionals know this. So why do they keep recommending minimal nutrient levels? Most are stuck in the past. They're still focused on deficiency diseases instead of thinking about what is required for optimum health.

What Has Happened to Today's Food?

To make matters worse, food today isn't what it used to be. One reason is that much of our modern diet consists of commercial foods that have been milled, refined, pasteurized, synthesized, and otherwise altered so that they are far from their natural state. Such processing often removes the vitamins, enzymes, fiber, and other nutrients that our bodies and brains need to function at peak performance levels. This includes the immune system, which protects you from infectious diseases and cancers, as well as your body's repair process, which heals damaged cells and tissues while slowing down the rate of aging.

Then there's the problem of commercial agriculture. One hundred years ago, American farmers were good stewards of the soil, returning to it the minerals and organic matter that keep it alive with bacteria and other beneficial microorganisms, which enrich plants with vitamins and nutrients. Not so today. After five decades of intensive chemicalized farming, most topsoil in the United States is inert dirt that produces crops containing just a fraction of the vitamins and minerals necessary for optimal health. Cooking depletes up to half of the nutrients that remain.

Plenty of studies show that the vitamin and mineral deficiencies in the foods we eat, along with our omission of nutritious foods, are among the main causes of most of today's serious ills, such as obesity, heart disease, diabetes, stroke, hypertension, and many others.

Some nutritional experts suggest that you should overhaul your entire diet if you want to become healthier. But few people are likely to make such radical changes. Nor do you have to. There is another way to reduce, or even eliminate, the health damage caused by poor nutrition. Adding a few key vitamins and supplements to your diet will replace the nutrients you're missing and help neutralize the harmful ingredients in some fast foods that cause inflammation in the body.

Persistent inflammation literally makes you older—measured not in calendar years, but in the risk of disease, disability, and premature death. Researchers are finding that inflammation (as indicated by an elevated C-reactive protein level) is one of the main causes not only of heart disease, but of almost every other serious illness, including Alzheimer's, arthritis, and cancer. The obvious solution is to reduce such inflammation in your body.

Simple dietary changes can make a huge difference. If you eat a lot of fast food, or dine out frequently, you'd do well to bump up the amounts of inflammation-fighting foods you eat at home, like fresh fruits, vegetables, berries, and fresh fish. But it's extremely difficult to get enough anti-inflammatory nutrients from our diets alone. And as I've mentioned earlier, most retail multivitamins contain relatively low doses per tablet or capsule.

For instance, the average multivitamin supplies about 60 milligrams of vitamin C. That's not even close to the amount needed to reduce inflammation in your arteries and joints and throughout your body. If you happen to smoke, or live with a smoker, or reside in an area where there is a lot of air pollution, that 60 mg. of vitamin C is going to be used up quickly. Your body can't battle inflammation on such a meager amount. Linus Pauling, the preeminent researcher on vitamin C, recommended that people "load up in the thousands of milligrams each day." While many have questioned the appropriateness of taking such mega-doses, there is no question in my mind that average fast-food-eating Americans need to get more vitamin C into their system.

The same is true of other important disease-fighting, inflammation-quelling nutrients. A multivitamin will give you partial protection, but it won't cover you all the way. Vitamin C, together with vitamins D and E—what I call the Big

Three—help neutralize much of the internal damage caused by fast food. Here's how.

How Free Radicals Age You

Many, if not most, of the serious diseases that strike North Americans are due to unstable oxygen molecules called free radicals. These are oxygen molecules that are missing an electron, which can get knocked off by chemical changes—from eating too much fat, for example. Since oxygen molecules don't like missing an electron, they look for replacements by zipping through the body like pinballs, snatching electrons from other molecules in the body's cells and thereby damaging them. Unfortunately, this electron theft creates even more free radicals. The longer this process continues, the more inflammation is generated in the body, harming more of its cells, tissues, and organs. This eventually leads to disease.

Your body has a natural defense against free radicals. It's an enzyme called *superoxide dismutase* (SOD) that possesses enough extra electrons to render the free radicals harmless. The problem is, your body has only a limited supply of this enzyme. If you eat a lot of fast food, thus creating a bumper crop of free radicals, your natural reserves of SOD decline. Once your supply is depleted, you are extremely vulnerable to inflammation and the diseases it can cause.

Antioxidants as Anti-Agers

This is where vitamins C and E come in. They're known as *antioxidants* because they perform the same job as SOD, donating extra oxygen electrons, which disarm free radicals. Vitamin C is among the most powerful antioxidants of them all. So if you love those burgers and fries, you'd better load up on it! A British study of more than 20,000 people found that those who consumed 109 mg. (which I consider low) or more of vitamin C daily cut their risk of death by 50 percent compared to those who got about half that amount. Evidence shows that larger quantities (up to a point) are even better. There's a good reason for this. Cholesterol, the gunky stuff that forms in your arteries, isn't harmful until free radicals get hold of it. They actually oxidize normal cholesterol, making it stick to artery walls. If you block the free radicals, you help protect the cholesterol. And that's exactly what vitamin C can do.

How much C do you need? If you eat a lot of fast food—or smoke—I'd strongly recommend taking a supplement that provides 250 to 500 mg. daily. This amount, combined with the vitamin C you get naturally from fruits, fruit juices, and vegetables, should put you in the safety zone.

Vitamin E is also a heart protector for those indulging in cheeseburgers and supersized shakes. Like C, vitamin E is extremely good at mopping up free radicals. But unlike vitamin C, which works in the watery parts of the body, vitamin E works in the fatty regions, protecting fatty tissues as well as your bloodstream. Vitamin E also makes cholesterol less likely to clog up your arteries. The Harvard Nurses' Health Study found that women with the highest vitamin E intake—about 200 IU a day—were a third less likely to develop heart disease than those getting much lower amounts.

Here are a couple more reasons to make friends with vitamin E. It has some blood-thinning capabilities that can prevent clots in the blood. It also makes the inner lining of your blood vessels act like Teflon, repelling any plaques that may want to cling to it. And if you should already have some fatty plaque deposits stuck in your arteries, vitamin E helps to stabilize them so they won't break off and cause a stroke or heart attack.

The official recommended daily dose for vitamin E is 30 IU. That's a joke. Plenty of studies show that you need much more to receive the protection I've just described. The tragedy is that the majority of people in the United States—especially people who eat a lot of fast food—don't even get that much. Little wonder we lead the world in heart disease.

My advice is to take a minimum of 100 to 200 IU of vitamin E daily. That's hard to achieve even when you're eating a healthy diet, so obviously you need a supplement. When shopping, look for vitamin E in the form of mixed tocopherols, including gamma-tocopherol and tocotrienols. This is the form that is most natural for the human body to assimilate. Just read the label or ask the store clerk or pharmacist for help.

I've already explained how most of us don't get enough vitamin D. Although not an antioxidant, vitamin D strengthens your immune system. In men, it protects the prostate gland from cancer. Many scientists believe that the high rates of prostate cancer in North America are strongly linked to insufficient vitamin D in the diet. In addition, many of the cancers that are linked to a high-fat diet, such as breast and colon cancer, can be prevented by simply making sure you get more vitamin D.

The most common source of vitamin D is sunshine. But the fear of skin cancer has led many people to avoid the sun altogether, or to apply so much sunscreen that the rays never penetrate to the skin. Ironically, these practices could be causing more cancers than they are preventing. True, you don't want to be overexposed, but you also don't want to run low on vitamin D. Experts recommend that you seek twenty minutes of unprotected sun daily.

What about a supplement? The official recommendation for vitamin D is 200 to 400 IU. I suggest taking at least 400 IU a day. Fortified breakfast cereals (when shopping, look for brands that are low in sugar and other sweeteners), milk, and fish are the best food sources. A cup of milk, for example, has 100 IU vitamin D. If you drink four cups a day, you should be fine, but most adults wouldn't want to consume that much milk and the extra calories that come with it. Spending about twenty minutes a day in the sun and taking a daily multivitamin that provides at least 400 IU vitamin D will properly protect you.

Mother Nature's Pharmacy

What other nutrients are especially important for frequent fast-food eaters? The Big Three are a good start, but equally important are compounds called *phytonutrients* that are abundant in plant foods. Many researchers now believe that these substances may play an even bigger role than vitamins in keeping us healthy—and in reversing any potential health damage from a fast-food diet.

Phytonutrients are beneficial chemicals found in plants. Think of them as Mother Nature's pharmacy, the good-for-you substances that are the reason doctors now recommend you eat at least five servings of fruits and vegetables every day to protect your body from heart disease, cancer, and other serious health problems.

Phytonutrients do some remarkable things in the human body. Take *lutein* and *zeaxanthin*. These two compounds are abundant in green leafy vegetables and are among the most powerful antioxidants ever discovered. Harvard researchers found that people whose diet contained more of these two substances lowered their risk of macular degeneration (a leading cause of blindness) by more than 40 percent. Wow! Any pharmaceutical company would be thrilled to have a new drug that produced such results. But this is an even better deal. You don't need a prescription; just eat more vegetables like spinach, broc-coli, and kale! While it is possible to find phytonutrient-rich foods at fast-food restaurants, you have to try harder. The amount of tomatoes and onions on a burger won't produce these dramatic results. Ditto for the salads. The best way to increase phytonutrients in your diet is to pack the produce drawers in your refrigerator with the brightest-colored fruits and vegetables you can find. They're the ones with the highest phytonutrient levels, and they can significantly reduce joint, muscle, and heart inflammation and protect your overall health.

I know what I'm about to say may sound difficult, but it really doesn't have to be. If you eat four to six fruit and veg-etable servings a day—as easy as grabbing an apple on the way out the door, munching a carrot at work, and having some extra vegetables at dinner—you'll be doing more for your health than a month's worth of doctor appointments.

Most North Americans, of course, don't eat anywhere near that many fruits and greens, so they are missing out on the benefits of phytonutrients. And don't believe the TV commer-cials for fruit juices. Store-bought fruit juices are loaded with excess calories and sugar that quickly become extra pounds—but not with phytonutrients. Fortunately, there are supplements available that can help make up the difference. They include:

Super sulfides   Order double onions the next time you choose a burger or a take-out taco—and don't forget to eat garlic at home. The same chemical compounds that bring tears to your eyes can save your life. Sound like an exaggeration? Not at all. A study of more than 120,000 people in the Netherlands found that those who consumed the most *allylic sulfides* (the medicinal compounds in these two foods) had the lowest rates of stomach cancer.

It gets better. In the kind of study I wish doctors would

conduct more often, volunteers were fed enough butter and lard to supply a small bakery. Then they were given a supplement made from onion extract. Not only did their cholesterol levels stay steady—remarkable when you consider how much fat they consumed—but clots in their blood dissolved more readily. And fewer clots mean less risk of heart attack and stroke.

As an Italian who loves to cook, I'd be lost without onions and garlic. Any cardiologist worth his salt should love them too for his patients' sake. They won't magically take inches off your waistline or undo years of dietary indiscretions, but they're among the few foods that can actually reverse some of the damage of high-fat eating.

Did you have a few fast-food meals this week? Make up for it at home by doubling or tripling the amount of onions and garlic you use in recipes. Another option is to take an odor-free garlic supplement that provides 500 mg. of allylic sulfides, which is more than enough. For suggestions for high-quality brands, check our free Web site, www.thefastfooddiet.com.

Carotenoids with clout   Here's another family of health-giving natural compounds that fast-food lovers should adopt. Research shows that the *carotenoids* (which include beta-carotene) have astonishing health benefits. These compounds decrease the risk of certain cancers, stroke, heart disease, and eye disease. Carotenoids also strengthen the immune system. They're found in many foods we eat (or should eat) every day, including cantaloupe, tomatoes, and all of the leafy vegetables—and yes, even some fast food.

Scientists are a long way from understanding *how* the carotenoids produce their wonderful benefits, but here are a few highlights of what we do know.

Lycopene   If you haven't been to Domino's or Papa John's or Pizza Hut lately, get in line! Pizza can be one of the best fast foods for you. Why? Because tomatoes (and especially tomato sauce) are jammed with *lycopene*, an antioxidant shown to slow down the growth of cancer cells. My wife used to joke that man's *real* best friend is a take-out pizza. And while I love our three dogs, medically speaking, she's correct. A five-year Harvard study of 48,000 men found that those who ate ten or more weekly servings of tomatoes and tomato sauce were two-thirds less likely to develop prostate cancer than men who ate only two servings. (One half of a tomato equals one serving.) Mexican salsa also counts. And get this: the ketchup on a burger or hot dog contains even more lycopene than fresh tomatoes.

Here's another fascinating finding. People who get a lot of carotenoids in their diets also have less risk of heart disease. Reason? Cholesterol and other oxidized gunk are less likely to stick to their artery walls. Besides that, their eyes stay healthier and their lenses remain sharper longer, with fewer occurrences of cataracts.

The fabulous flavonoids   This is another group of plant chemicals dear to my cardiological heart. I won't bore you with all of the scientific details, but here's the short version. *Flavonoids* are powerful antioxidants that help reduce inflammation in the arteries. They also make blood cells more slippery so they are less likely to clump together and form clots. Abundant in red wine (along with apples, onions, celery, grapes, and even tea), flavonoids are thought to be the reason that the butter-loving, cigarette-smoking French have only a fraction of the heart-disease rates that North Americans do. We doctors call this the "French Paradox."

But we are not alone in this. A study of more than five

thousand Finns found that those who got the fewest flavonoids in their diets had the highest risk of heart disease. The best news is that you don't need a lot of flavonoids to reap the benefits. In a Dutch study, people who ate as little as half an apple or an eighth of a cup of onions, or drank four cups of tea a day, were a third less likely to die from heart attacks than those who got fewer flavonoids in their diets.

Flavonoids have also aroused considerable interest recently because of their potential beneficial effects as antivirals and anti-allergics with antiplatelet and antitumor properties.

If you're taking a multivitamin, look for one that contains at least 25 milligrams of a substance called *quercetin*. This is the flavonoid that's been most widely studied—and appears to have the most powerful effects. A glass of red wine while dining out? It's good medicine!

Incredible isothiocyanates   Woo-eee—what's that smell? If you've ever cooked broccoli, Brussels sprouts, or cabbage, you know they can really perfume the house. But please don't let the strong smell discourage you. What you're sniffing are some of the most remarkable plant medicines on earth. All cruciferous vegetables contain compounds called *isothiocyanates*. One type, *sulforaphane*, is a nutrient that neutralizes harmful chemicals *before* they can initiate the cancer-causing process.

I realize that a lot of people don't particularly love cooking crucifers. So make life easy for yourself and let someone else prepare them. Get a pizza that includes broccoli, or order a cauliflower side at your favorite steak house. A couple of servings of crucifers a week can offset a lot of the potential damage done by fast-food fat and other unhealthy ingredients.

The Powerhouse B's

I've talked a lot about eliminating (or at least reducing) the onslaught of free-radical molecules. The B vitamins are among the most powerful nutrients that can clean up their damage. New research also indicates that the B's quell inflammation from fast food and other causes. Unless you eat the kind of diet that would do a nutritionist proud, my advice is to make sure you take a B-complex supplement containing 400 to 800 mcg. of folate, along with 100 percent of the recommend daily amounts of vitamins B_6 and B_{12}. Here's why.

Folate   Earlier I mentioned folate's role in suppressing DNA damage that can lead to cancer. But there's another reason to get more folate than the official recommendation: it significantly lowers levels of a nasty chemical called *homocysteine*, which causes massive amounts of inflammation in the arteries (leading to heart disease) and in the brain (resulting in poor memory, dementia, and Alzheimer's disease).

Studies show that elevated homocysteine in your blood doubles your risk of heart attack and stroke, because it scars and burns the inner lining of blood vessels. There's good evidence that people who lower homocysteine by getting sufficient folate live longer and suffer fewer of these diseases.

If you eat a lot of fast food—or for that matter, a lot of rich, fatty home cooking—folate is one nutrient you need more of. All sorts of foods, including beans and fortified cereals, contain some folate, but not enough to hit the optimal levels. That's why I recommend supplements, which are also more readily absorbed by the body than the folate in foods. Look for a B-complex supplement that contains all of the B vitamins along with at least 400 mcg. of folate.

Vitamins B_6 and B_{12} If you're boosting your levels of folate, you'll also need to take vitamins B_6 and B_{12}, because they are necessary for folate to work efficiently. Vitamin B_6 is also helpful to people with carpal tunnel syndrome and to diabetics with the eye disease called *retinopathy*. Since fast food is closely linked to Type 2 diabetes, it makes sense to protect your eyes with vitamin B_6. I recommend it to all of my patients. The recommended daily dose is just 2 mg., which is about right for most people. That's the amount you'll find included in most multi- and B-complex supplements. But it certainly wouldn't hurt to get a little more— about 10 mg. per day—if you're fifty-five years or older, since that's around the time that the human body starts absorbing less B_6. If you are concerned with your body's ability to absorb B_6, add peridoxal-5-phosphate (P5P) to your daily supplement regime. The body transforms P5P into a highly absorbable form of B_6.

Vitamin B_{12} acts similarly to B_6 and folate—only better. A number of studies have shown that many older adults, including those with Alzheimer's disease, are deficient in B_{12}. Low levels of B_{12} are a common cause of memory problems, and it's easy to confuse a simple nutritional deficiency with something more serious.

Nearly all of us get enough vitamin B_{12} in our diet (it's found in eggs, meats, and other animal foods), but as with B_6, absorption can plummet in older adults. I suggest you take a multi- or B-complex supplement that provides more than 100 percent of the recommended daily amount (RDA) of vitamin B_{12}. I take 100 mcg. daily. You'll wind up with more because so many foods, especially meats, contain healthy amounts. Vegetarians must take a supplement to get enough B_{12}.

Fantastic Fish Oil

Here are two statistics that might knock your socks off. The average North American consumes about 120 mg. a day of DHA (one of the natural oils in fish). And we have the highest incidence of cancer in the world. On the other hand, the average Japanese consumes about 600 mg. of the same oil and Japan has the world's lowest cancer rate. Coincidence? Hardly.

Plenty of solid scientific evidence shows that fish and fish oils are among the healthiest foods on the planet. In fact, boosting your intake of fish and/or fish oil supplements can almost erase the nutritional damage caused by years (or a lifetime) of unhealthy eating. Of course, there's no substitute for an all-around good diet, and someone who lives on fast food all week isn't likely to win the World's Healthiest Person award. DHA and other fish oils work directly in the arteries and other parts of the body to reduce inflammation, prevent many diseases, and extend your life. Here's what happens if your fish oil consumption is low.

- When you eat a diet high in saturated fat or trans fat—the typical North American diet, in other words—the fat is oxidized in your arteries and turns rancid.

- This oxidized fat generates enormous quantities of free radicals.

- The free radicals enhance the damage done by *arachidonic acid*, a dangerous inflammatory chemical.

- The resulting inflammation causes damaged arteries, blood clots, neurological diseases, and so on.

This unfortunate situation can be reversed by eating two or three fish meals a week—including the broiled fish available at most restaurants. (Fried fish doesn't count because frying destroys the health benefits.) Fish oils are pure gold for your heart, especially if you eat a lot of fast food. Unfortunately, many people don't like fish. They don't know how to prepare it properly. They don't like the smell. Or they simply dislike the taste. So what to do?

Fish oil supplements are the easy solution. In fact, some research shows that fish oil capsules provide more health benefits than fish itself. Nowadays, species such as shark, swordfish, big tuna, halibut, and grouper are known to accumulate dangerous levels of mercury in their tissues and should be avoided. If you don't eat fish very often (or at all), I suggest you take a daily supplement containing 1,000 mg. of fish oil. If you have high blood pressure, take even more; as much as 2,000 to 3,000 mg.

An alternative to fish oil capsules are a couple of tablespoons of crushed flaxseed every day. You can sprinkle it on your morning cereal, on your cottage cheese at lunch, or on top of evening salads. Adding a small amount of olive oil to your cottage cheese or salad in addition to flaxseed will increase its effectiveness. Flaxseed is tasty enough to also eat it by the spoonful. It is loaded with *alpha-linolenic acid*, a substance that's converted in the body into omega-3 fatty acid, which is what makes fish oil so good for your heart and arteries.

Stay Fit with Fiber

Just about everyone has heard how important fiber is for good health. It benefits the heart and arteries. It lowers cholesterol. It improves digestion. Some research even shows that it helps reduce the risk of cancer. With so much going for it, you'd think that people would eat more fiber. But they don't. The average North American gets only about 11 or 12 grams of fiber a day. That's nowhere close to the 30 to 40 grams needed for optimal health.

Why do we eat so little? Mostly because we have grown up on the traditional American diet, which includes lots of meat, plenty of starchy carbohydrates, and relatively few "whole" foods—fruits, vegetables, whole grains, and beans. Our taste buds never learned to appreciate plant foods. Though Mom tried to get us to eat our veggies, most of us found them too "yucky."

But there's no way around the fact that you must include more fiber into your diet to minimize the damage caused by munching down too many fast foods. Fiber in plant foods helps by sponging up cholesterol molecules in the intestine and eliminating them from the body. And by now, we all know that lowering cholesterol is one way to cut the risk of heart disease. Fiber also absorbs bile acids and other potential carcinogens. At the same time, it causes the stool to move through the bowel more quickly. This is important because the less time fats, cholesterol, and carcinogens spend in the intestine, the less likely they are to find their way back into the bloodstream, where they can cause artery disease, cancer, inflammation, and other health problems.

Then there's the diabetes link. If you've eaten a lot of fast food in your life and have managed to pack on some extra weight, your risk of developing diabetes is higher than the average person's. Fiber can help you reverse this danger because it slows the absorption of glucose into the blood and minimizes its "spikes," which stimulate appetite and increase your risk of both more weight gain and full-fledged diabetes. In landmark research sponsored by the Diabetes Prevention Program, doctors discovered that a healthful, fiber-filled diet—combined with weight loss and exercise—reduced the risk of diabetes by 58 percent. Participants in the study lost an average of 15 pounds by eating more fiber and consuming just 450 fewer calories a day. That's pretty painless. Here are some easy ways to get more fiber into your diet.

- The best natural way to increase fiber consumption is to eat a lot of fruit, produce, whole grains, and beans each and every day. The more plant foods you eat, the more fiber you get.

- Oatmeal and oat bran are terrific sources of fiber—and the type they contain (soluble fiber) is ideal for cholesterol control.

- There's nothing wrong with using a fiber supplement to bump up your intake. I often advise patients to take a few daily tablespoons of Metamucil. It's made with *psyllium*, a seed that is one of Mother Nature's most concentrated fiber sources. Crushed flaxseed is another superb source of fiber, which also provides your body with omega-3 fatty acids at the same time.

The Magic Minerals

Calcium, magnesium, and potassium are the most important minerals for people who eat a lot of fast food. Why? Because they help to keep blood pressure and heart rhythms in the safety zone. For instance:

Calcium   If you're taking a multivitamin that doesn't include at least 500 mg. of calcium, toss out the bottle and buy one that does. Or at least buy a calcium-only supplement. This is especially important if you drink a lot of soft drinks, which contain *phosphoric acid*, which pulls calcium out of your bones faster than you can imagine. This easily leads to the brittle bone condition known as osteoporosis.

I used to coach Midget League football. One year, I noticed that a lot of my guys were sustaining bone fractures. It finally dawned on me that these eleven-, twelve-, and thirteen-year-old boys owned fracture-prone bones because

The Anti-Diabetes Mineral

Chromium is a trace mineral that the body utilizes to break down simple sugar and carbohydrates, among other things. It's called a "trace" mineral because you need only about 120 micrograms (mcg.) daily. But just because you need only a small amount, don't underestimate its importance. Without chromium, you are extremely vulnerable to developing diabetes. And many people in developed countries simply aren't getting enough of this mineral because it is largely absent in highly processed, agriculturally depleted foods—especially fast foods.

A deficiency of chromium can lead to insulin resistance, a major risk factor for diabetes. Quite a few medical studies show that people with diabetes who take chromium supplements achieve better blood-sugar control. In some cases, they're able to reduce their dosage of medication.

Most chromium supplements come in 200 mcg. tablets. Doctors usually recommend taking them one to three times daily. *Important*: For optimal absorption, drink a glass of orange juice with your chromium because vitamin C improves its absorption by the body.

they were gulping down too many soft drinks. They had the type of bones doctors see in postmenopausal women!

Speaking of postmenopause, women should start supplementing with calcium early in life to protect their bones. And if you eat a rich diet—heavy on meat and light on dairy or plant foods—make sure you get extra calcium, because it can help protect your heart. There's also good evidence that calcium can lower your blood pressure into a healthier range. Women who haven't reached menopause need 1,000 mg. daily, and postmenopausal women should get 1,500 mg. Men should take 500 mg. of calcium a day. Just make sure you stick to small doses, because the human body (male or female) can only utilize about 500 mg. at a time. Calcium should only be taken after meals.

Potassium This is another one of those minerals that few people seem to take seriously. But of all of them, potassium is among the most important minerals for controlling blood pressure and preventing heart problems. Considering our high-fat, high-salt, and high-cholesterol diets, getting enough potassium isn't optional; it's a must. Here's why.

Nearly all North Americans eat way too much salt, and this is especially true for fast-food consumers. All that salt concentrates in the blood and causes your body to dilute it with fluids. (That's why salty foods make you thirsty.) When you drink more liquids, your body retains them and the amount of fluid in your bloodstream rises, causing your blood pressure to shoot up. Potassium helps to relieve the problem by promoting the excretion of sodium so your blood pressure can return to normal. This is a good thing because lowering blood pressure can save your life. A Harvard study found that people with the lowest intake of potassium (an average of 2,000 mg. a day) had the greatest risk of stroke. In addition to getting rid of excess salt, potassium also relaxes the blood vessels and promotes better circulation—another key to lowering blood pressure.

I recommend 3,500 mg. of potassium daily for everyone. It's not hard to do, even if you dine out a lot. One baked potato delivers 844 mg. of potassium. A serving of yogurt has nearly 500 mg. And one banana contains 467 mg. Dried fruits are another great source of potassium, though they are high in calories.

Magnesium   This amazing mineral acts like a drug in protecting the heart. Patients with angina (chest pain due to insufficient blood supply) have been successfully treated with nothing more than magnesium. It has been shown to save lives when taken shortly after a heart attack. It also helps normalize irregular heart rhythms (arrhythmias), which can be potentially fatal. And, like potassium, it has the ability to lower blood pressure.

Foods naturally rich in magnesium are tofu, figs, kelp (a type of seaweed), and pumpkin seeds. Admittedly, these may not be the kinds of foods most people have in their kitchen cabinets. Other options include brown rice, spinach, oatmeal, and beans.

Your body needs only about 400 mg. of magnesium a day. Most multivitamins contain anywhere from 100 to 200 mg. So if you take a daily supplement and also cook up some nutritious, magnesium-rich foods, you'll easily take in enough.

If you're overweight, you should definitely supplement with magnesium, because it has been shown to reduce the risk of insulin resistance, a condition that often precedes full-blown diabetes. There's also evidence that magnesium can help reduce abdominal fat, especially in postmenopausal women, a key risk factor for heart disease.

CHAPTER 11

The Fast-Food Diet for Business Travelers

Pity the poor traveler. Especially the business traveler. Our nation's airports are the perfect places for making people fat. Start with two million Americans who fly every day. Throw in unpredictable schedules and late flights to guarantee that lots of bored, stressed people will be stuck for hours in the airport. Then make food the main entertainment, with mall-like food courts and plenty of fast-food restaurants. Even after travelers board their flights, the airlines use snack foods and alcohol to make them forget that they're traveling at six hundred miles per hour in a metal tube five miles above the ground.

If you spend much time traveling by air, it's almost impossible to avoid a terminal collision with some of today's most fattening foods. The nation's biggest airports feature the same fast-food restaurants that play a key role in America's ever-expanding waistlines everywhere else. While you're waiting

Fly the Less-Flabby Skies

It's easy enough to find fat-filled, sugar-packed, calorie-loaded snacks and meals at our nation's airports. But it's also getting easier to find healthful, low-carb meals. A survey conducted by the Physicians Committee for Responsible Medicine identified twelve of the nation's busiest airports that offer the most nutritious food. Restaurants made the grade if they served at least one breakfast, lunch, or supper that's low in fat, high in fiber, and cholesterol-free. Each airport was scored on the percentage of healthful restaurants among the total restaurants available.

1. Miami International Airport, 85 percent
2. Detroit Metropolitan Airport, 83 percent
3. Denver International Airport, 78 percent
4. Chicago O'Hare International Airport, 75 percent
5. John F. Kennedy International Airport (New York), 73 percent
6. Hartsfield-Jackson Atlanta International Airport, 64 percent
7. Newark Liberty International Airport, 63 percent
8. Dallas/Fort Worth International Airport, 59 percent
9. Minneapolis-St. Paul International Airport, 54 percent
10. Los Angeles International Airport, 53 percent
11. Phoenix Sky Harbor International Airport, 44 percent
12. McCarran International Airport (Las Vegas), 33 percent

for your flight, you can drop in at McDonald's, Burger King, Panda Express, or The Cheesecake Factory, among others. You can choose from softball-sized muffins and pastries, such as the 1,100-calorie Pecanbon at Cinnabon, Mrs. Fields's 270-calorie White Chunk Macadamia Cookie, or Auntie Anne's 510-calorie Glazin' Raisin Pretzel with butter.

With choices like these, it's obvious why frequent fliers weigh more than they used to. It's easy to chomp down 500 to 1,000 calories on the snacks alone. Throw in a meal at one of the chains and you'll waddle home a few pounds heavier than when you said farewell to your family.

Airports are finally getting the hint that people want leaner choices. A survey by the American Dietetic Association of twenty-eight major airports reports that it is (finally!) becoming easier to eat nutritiously and cut back on calories while waiting for a flight. Detroit's Metropolitan Airport partnered with Henry Ford Health System to encourage restaurants to improve their offerings. They also launched their Heart Smart program, in which participating restaurants use a red logo to indicate healthier choices. Other airports are in hot pursuit. It's still not easy to find great food, but at least now it's possible to come home with the same amount of baggage you left with. Here are some weight-friendly travel tips.

Snack lightly   There's a saying in the travel business: "Vacation food has no calories." That means it's pretty easy to abandon your diet and your good intentions when traveling away from home. No big deal if you only travel once or twice a year, but it's a real trap for frequent fliers. My advice: Don't use up a day's calories on snacks. When your stomach's growling, have some mixed nuts. Or get a fruit cup, an apple, or a container of yogurt. Save the "blow-out" calories for a meal you'll really enjoy. Cutting down on high-calorie airport snacks could eliminate quite a few extra pounds in a year.

Settle your stomach with a smoothie   Just about every airport has a smoothie or yogurt franchise. If you order something low on the fat-and-calorie scale, you won't have to worry about your weight. Better yet, if you order a smoothie with low-fat milk or yogurt, you'll get enough lean protein to set-tle your stomach for the next few hours, along with an extra fruit serving for the day. The 20-ounce Berry Slim Smoothie at TCBY, for example, only has 300 calories—410 if you get it with yogurt.

Check out the salad and eggs   Quite a few of the airport chains offer green salads as well as hard-boiled eggs. It's an almost perfect combination. The salad has very few calories (as long as you go easy on the dressing), and the fat and protein in the eggs are supreme for holding your appetite in check because they help control insulin levels.

Eat hearty, eat light   If you have time for a sit-down meal, take advantage of some of the newer, healthier airport chains. Mediterranean Grill has an excellent high-fiber, low-fat menu, including such menu items as tabbouleh and chicken stir-fry. Panda Express, the largest of the food-court chains, also makes it easier to order a weight-control meal, especially if you get a side of rice and an all-vegetable entrée. Or check out the Online Café Bar and Grill, which includes diet-perfect entrées such as a vegetarian sandwich and smoked turkey spinach wrap.

Chugalug the water   It's easy to get dehydrated when you fly, so drinking extra water is essential. It's also a good way to keep your weight in check. Weight-loss experts have found that people often confuse thirst for hunger. When you're starting to feel those early pangs, slug down a bottle. You might find that you weren't all that hungry to begin with—and even if you are, drinking water first will reduce the amount of calories you need to feel satisfied.

Order ahead   Meals are rarely served to coach-class passen-gers anymore, but they're standard in first class and busi-ness class. Yet airline food is no more likely to be low in fat or calories than it is to be tasty. Give yourself a break and order a healthier meal—vegetarian, kosher, or low-calorie—when you make your reservation. These are often fresher and of better quality because they are prepared on board. If you do order after take-off, choose something that's high in protein (like chicken or beef). It will hold your appetite and maintain insulin control better than a high-carb meal. Incidentally, even if you didn't order ahead for a special meal, ask for one. There's a chance you'll get it, because the airline may keep a few extras on hand.

Pack your own   Why depend on mediocre airport food when you can just as easily pack your own snack: a few pieces of fruit, a Baggie-full of unsalted almonds or trail mix, or a yogurt cup? The idea isn't to live like a Spartan and give up great food once you reach your destination. Rather, it's to reduce those "mindless" calories that keep you busy in transit. Save yourself for meals you'll really enjoy.

Stop and Go: Calorie Control at the Convenience Store

Of course, flying isn't the only way to travel. Many of us prefer to pack up the van and head for the great open road for our vacation. This can be loads of fun, provided we pack the right food and beverages. If we don't, we usually find ourselves bored, tired, hungry, and at the mercy of the snack food section of some off-the-interstate gas station. And that can be a wrong turn for your waistline.

Have you ever walked into a convenience store or gas station, made the purchase you intended to make, and walked out with all of your change still in your pocket? I didn't think so. Those stores are brilliantly designed to tempt you with hundreds of impulse purchases. The food selection at convenience stores and gas stations can rival the choices at a well-stocked neighborhood market. The only difference is that convenience store fare is more likely to cost you an extra 250, 500, or 1,000 calories. And all you really wanted was a newspaper, a gallon of milk, or a tank of gas. What makes these places really dangerous is that you can easily eat up 25 percent or more of your daily calorie budget just by ripping into a small snack. Check the label on Dolly's Zingers vanilla cream-filled cakes. In a couple of bites you'll down 470 calories and 15 grams of fat. A Snickers bar doesn't last even as long as the cakes, but it has a scary 280 calories and 14 grams of fat.

The prepared foods aren't necessarily any better. For example, the Ham and Cheese Bagel Melt at Wawa packs 485 calories and 13 grams of fat (including 7 grams of saturated fat). The Turkey American Pretzel Melt is in the same league, with 440 calories and 16 grams of fat. Eat one of those every day for a year and you could easily gain 45 pounds or more!

Convenience stores have become part of our culinary landscape because there are always times when you're hungry, in a hurry, and in need of something quick. While it's not possible to get great food at these stops, you can choose *okay* food that won't totally blow your diet. Here are some tips to guide you through the junk food jungle.

Snack lightly   Snacks are important when you're trying to lose weight, because they keep your hunger under control. If you wait too long before eating, you'll become ravenous and want to eat everything in sight. What types of snacks are best? If you lived on a remote mountain in the middle of Crete or somewhere in China, a normal snack might be the handful of nuts or the piece of fruit you'd find right around you; that's ideal. But here in America, this isn't always

Beyond the Vending Machine

Snacking between meals isn't a guilty pleasure. It's a practical way to manage your hunger, keep your blood sugar and insulin stable, limit your overall calorie intake, and accelerate your body's ability to burn fat instead of storing it. Yet most of the snacks that are readily available are precisely the ones that make it almost impossible to lose weight. For example, just one package with two Reese's Peanut Butter Cups has 280 calories and 17 grams of fat. Think those cheese-filled crackers are better? Not by much. Eat a couple of vending-machine snacks and you're looking at about a *third* of a woman's calorie budget for an entire day.

Even if you're not a super-organized person, make it a point to pack your own snacks. When you can't, look for these commercial ones that won't overload your diet with fat and calories. For instance:

- **Crunchy Peanut Butter Clif Bar**   It's sweet enough to satisfy any sugar craving, but is relatively light on calories (240) and provides 5 grams of fiber.

- **Planters Honey-Roasted Cashews**   They're somewhat high in fat, but most of the fat is the heart-healthy monounsaturated kind. At 230 calories, this is a vending-machine snack you can live with.

- **Dannon Light 'n Fit with Fiber Strawberry Yogurt**   It has zero fat, almost zero cholesterol, and only 70 calories. Plus, it packs 3 grams of fiber.

- **Kraft Handi Snacks Mozzarella String Cheese**   These 1-ounce, bite-sized snacks aren't exactly fat-free, but with only 80 calories, they'll do. Besides, the fat and protein will settle your stomach and keep you from getting hungry twenty minutes later.

possible. When your snack tooth is raging, try to minimize the dietary damage by picking something that isn't loaded with processed sugar and fat, such as a cup of yogurt, a bag of nuts or trail mix, dried fruit, or a slice of beef jerky.

Shoot for 250 calories   That's the limit for a perfect snack. Once a snack gets into the 500-calorie range, you're looking more at a small meal. This can represent a third of the calories the average woman needs for the entire day and a quarter of the calories for the average man. Snack smart.

Get a whole-food sandwich   Many of the hot and cold hoagies at convenience stores can be lean and nutritious. A good rule is to avoid sandwiches loaded with cheese or processed dressings. The typical turkey on whole wheat has barely 300 calories with less than 3 grams of fat. A ham-on-kaiser is only a little richer, with 337 calories and 6 grams of fat. A hot dog with chili and cheese sauce? Fagetaboutit!

Check out the produce   Most convenience stores and gas stations offer at least one fruit or veggie snack. That's not always what you're craving when the Snack Beast strikes, but with almost no calories or fat, plus plenty of fiber and antioxidants, it's a good way to take the edge off your appetite if you're serious about losing weight.

Drink some tea   A surprising number of the calories in the North American diet come in a bottle. Sodas are the worst offenders, but sweetened fruit drinks aren't far behind. Bottled iced tea is a better choice, as long as you aren't bothered by the caffeine. Buy the unsweetened kind, the one without high fructose corn syrup or artificial sweeteners. It won't put a dent in your calorie limit and you'll get loads of heart-healthy antioxidants at the same time.

CHAPTER 12

The Fast-Food Diet
for the Holidays

It's tough enough to lose weight under normal circumstances, but it's a real bear during the holidays. Discipline and motivation seem to be the first casualties when we put on our party hats. It's not just the sheer amount of cookies, fudge, brownies, and candies that appear between October and January. It's the fact that we're all socializing a lot more than usual. There are office parties, sumptuous feasts with friends, and happy hours that never seem to end. With all of those delectable calories up for grabs, it's not surprising that most people gain at least a couple of pounds or more.

I'd never advise anyone to become a holiday hermit just to avoid a few caloric indiscretions. Nor does it make sense for anyone to deprive themselves of traditional holiday spreads. Turkey with all the trimmings is too good to resist. Come to think of it, so is the rum and eggnog. Then there are the boxes of holiday cookies that arrive in the mail, and the lavish office parties where everyone finally gets to let their hair down. These are the kinds of things that make the holidays special, so enjoy them!

At the same time, remember that pounds gained during the holidays don't automatically evaporate after New Year's. The trick is to enjoy the festivities without carrying around the weighty consequences until Labor Day—or beyond. Here are a few ideas.

Abandon the "starve and feast" approach   This is a common strategy among people who try to control their holiday calories. "If I skip breakfast or lunch," they think, "the extra calories eaten at parties won't make a difference." But this never works. Studies show that meal-skippers actually tend to take in *more* calories overall. Worse, your metabolism drops when you go hungry, so your body stores and hoards fat. *It's better to stick to your regular schedule.* Eat your usual breakfast and lunch. Have a snack or two during the day. You don't want to be starving when you sit down to a holiday spread or get within striking distance of a buffet.

Remember the optimal balance   The most effective weight-loss diet is one that includes 25 to 30 percent lean protein, 25 to 30 percent healthy fats, and 45 to 50 percent low-glycemic carbohydrates. People who strike this balance store less fat, burn more calories, and feel better overall than those who binge on (or shun) particular foods. Equally important, these wise folks can sample everything on the holiday table without feeling as if their "diet" is pulling them down. So help yourself to the turkey. It's a top-flight source of protein. Dig into the sweet potatoes and veggies for slow-burning, low-glycemic carbs. Get your fill of healthy fats from appetizer olives, fish entrées, or splashes of olive oil on your vegetables. Once you've done that, have some dessert. As long as you maintain the optimal carb-protein-fat balance, and keep your portions in a reasonable range, the calories will pretty much take care of themselves.

Limit the libations   It's easy to forget that the drink in your hand, plus the one before and the one after, can pack as many calories as a good-sized serving of chocolate mousse. As an extra whammy, alcohol also makes people hungrier and lowers their inhibitions, so they're more likely to gorge. A glass or two of wine with dinner won't blow your diet—and, in fact, doctors say it's good for your overall health. But only if you stop there. Keep drinking, and you risk crashing your diet, along with the party.

Eat early, party late   One of the most effective ways to limit holiday calories is to eat a little something before you go to the party. Slather a wheat cracker with peanut butter. Munch an apple. Grab a handful of nuts. Don't eat so much that you can't enjoy the food to come; just snack enough to take the edge off your appetite. Combining a low-glycemic carbohydrate with a healthy fat and protein, like the whole-grain cracker with peanut butter, is particularly good because it stabilizes blood sugar and controls your appetite for two to four hours.

Divide and conquer   Sweets and rich appetizers are everywhere during the holidays—and all those little somethings added together can load your system with more calories than the main meals. You needn't deprive yourself of anything, just cut back your portions a little. Fill three-quarters of your plate with healthier food and use the remaining quarter for the "indulgences." This kind of compromise lets you enjoy everything without paying a weighty price later.

Eat what you love   When researchers ask people what went wrong when they failed to lose weight on a particular diet, the word "deprivation" always tops the list. None of us is willing to give up the foods we truly love, at least not for long. My advice is: Don't say no to anything—and don't settle for second-best. Why choose the pumpkin pie (which you might not love) just because it has fewer calories than the pecan pie (which you adore)? Feel free to eat what you like. Sure, you might swallow a little more fat and calories than you planned. But if you stop with one piece and eat a little leaner the next day, it will all balance out. Remember the 80/20 Rule—and enjoy your 20 percent to the max!

Alternate feast days with regular days   The year-end holidays aren't over in a day or a week; they go on for months. And a lot of people give themselves "party permission" to live it up for the duration. Over the course of the holiday season, that can add up to a heck of a lot of extra calories. Here's a smarter approach: Set aside three or four days a week during which you'll go easy on red meat, fast food, or other things that run high in the fat and calorie department. Mainly stick with whole grains, bean salads, vegetable-spiked green salads, and other good-for-your-weight foods. The rest of the days, allow yourself to cut loose a little with richer (but still sensible) restaurant meals, fast food, or desserts. This approach gives you the best of both worlds: living "large" when you're inclined to, but without winding up larger in the New Year.

CHAPTER 13

The Fast-Food Diet for Vegetarians

I t's remarkable how quickly vegetarian eating has become part of the mainstream American diet. As recently as the 1980s, people who identified themselves as vegetarians were generally derided as being part of the "crunchy granola crowd." These days, just about everyone knows someone who's a vegetarian—and even people who aren't purists are often happy to go meatless every now and then. A National Restaurant Association poll reported that about 20 percent of Americans *at least occasionally* look for vegetarian meals when they dine out.

Study after study shows that people who increase their consumption of plant foods, while decreasing intake of meat, have lower cholesterol and blood pressure, and much lower risks for cancer, heart disease, and stroke. Plant foods are also ideal for weight control (or loss) because they are high in fiber, low in fat, and generally high in low-glycemic carbohydrates. They supply plant chemicals, which protect the body's cells and tissues from the cascade of destruction that has been linked to many of our most serious chronic diseases.

Still, relatively few North Americans are willing to give up meat altogether. Unless you live in one of the larger cities, you're unlikely to find more than a few (if any) restaurants that devote all or most of their menus to vegetarian dishes. This leaves those restaurant chains, which have stepped up to the plate, little to build on. Many offer just one or two meatless entrées, along with a somewhat greater selection of side dishes.

The Meatless Challenge

If your interest in going meatless is primarily about weight loss, don't assume that a vegetarian dish is necessarily lower in fat or calories. A veggie sandwich can be loaded with more calories or saturated fat than a Whopper! The cheese alone can add a few hundred calories to any dish. Even without the cheese, dishes often arrive drenched in butter, margarine, or trans fat. Salad dressings are among the main calorie offenders. So are baked goods, which can have more fat and calories than an equal serving of red meat.

Meatless meals at restaurants pose a couple of challenges. They have to be filling and tasty enough so you feel you're getting your money's worth, yet low enough in fat and calories to keep your weight where you want it. You have to know what to look for—and what to ask for.

Fast food for vegetarians   Nearly all of the fast-food chains offer at least one vegetarian dish, and some offer more. Yet the choices at these chains are limited. You can certainly get side dishes that fall into the vegetarian category, but main meals? Not much there.

- **Wendy's**   It offers a variety of packaged salads, along with baked potatoes and pitas, both with a choice of fillings.

- **Taco Bell**   Well, there's the Bean Burrito. Ask for it with salsa to zip up the flavor.

- **McDonald's**   You can get a fruit cup or a salad, but that's about it.

- **Subway**   This is about your best choice for fast-food vegetarian. You can order a sub that's smothered in veggies and low-fat toppings, all on a whole-grain roll.

- **Pizza Hut**   Actually, any pizza chain is a good choice for the vegetarian because you can pick your toppings and go easy on the cheese.

- **Burger King**   Hats off to this brave franchise for offering the BK Veggie Burger. Made from a blend of grains and fresh vegetables and topped with the usual fixings, it's big enough to be a meal in itself—and with 420 calories and only 3 grams of saturated fat, it's a good choice both for calorie control and long-term health.

Eat ethnic   Since much of the world's population eats less meat than Westerners do, it's easier to find stomach-satisfying vegetarian meals at ethnic restaurants than at traditional restaurant chains. Any Asian restaurant will offer a good selection of vegetable and tofu dishes, often served with rice or noodles. But be careful at typical Chinese restaurants; they often go heavy on the fats. At Indian restaurants, the dal (a dish made with curried lentils) is a popular vegetarian choice. Just about any ethnic restaurant, with the exception of Mexican, usually offers half a dozen or more vegetarian entrées and sides.

Bypass the entrées   The most dependable way to eat a vegetarian meal at most American restaurants is to order a variety of side dishes: mashed potatoes, corn, string beans, pasta salad, and so on. These dishes aren't always low in fat or calories, however, unless you ask the chef to hold the butter, oil, and rich sauces. Most of them are happy to accommodate you.

Give the chains a chance   More and more sit-down restaurants are expanding the meatless parts of their menus. If you haven't checked out the vegetarian offerings in a few years, you might be pleasantly surprised.

- P.F. Chang's has among the best vegetarian menu, with creative and filling dishes ranging from Shanghai Cucumbers and Sichuan Style Asparagus to Stir-Fried Spicy Eggplant. Most of these dishes are low in calories as well as saturated fat.

- Chili's features a Guiltless Black Bean Burger that's as juicy as any burger on the menu. With 650 calories and 2 grams of saturated fat, it's about as healthy as you can get and still use the name "burger."

- T.G.I. Friday's offers a number of vegan and vegetarian dishes, including the Gardenburger and a vegetable baguette, which can be ordered without cheese. They also serve vegetable-stuffed baked potatoes, and Chinese noodles in a spicy peanut sauce.

I singled out a few of the chains above, but you can do pretty well at just about any sit-down restaurant if you special-order. Most establishments will go out of their way to make you happy, even if this means serving a chicken salad without the chicken, adding extra vegetables to a stir-fry that usually comes with meat, or including other goodies to round out your meatless meal.

CHAPTER 14

The Fast-Food Diet Walking Plan

Walking used to be the Rodney Dangerfield of the exercise world; it got no respect. But all that suddenly changed when scientists started looking at the numbers. New research suggests that walking may be the most effective form of exercise there is (not to mention, the safest). Here's why: Walking burns an average of 100 calories per mile. If you walk for an hour most days of the week, you'll lose about four pounds a month—even if you never change your diet one iota. This hour a day of walking will add about five years to your life span. It promotes steady weight loss, improves cardiovascular conditioning, and reduces the risk of diabetes.

The medical fact is, the more vigorous forms of exercise, such as jogging or working out in a gym, don't provide any additional health benefits—but greatly increase the risk of damage to your muscles, bones, joints, or heart.

A few years ago, McDonald's teamed up with exercise

Bet on the METs

It's hardly news that regular exercise promotes good cardiovascular health. But new studies indicate that the best heart protection occurs at higher levels of oxygen use than previously thought.

A measure of aerobic fitness called METs (metabolic equivalents) appears to be one of the most powerful predictors of heart and blood vessel health. Walking at a leisurely pace uses about three METs. Very brisk walking uses about eight. A previously sedentary adult who increases MET capacity from five to eight (or higher) could reduce the risk of dying from heart disease by 30 to 40 percent.

Increasing METs lowers heart rate and blood pressure, improves the body's sensitivity to insulin (meaning it can produce less of this fat-storing hormone), improves cholesterol, and inhibits the formation of clots, the cause of most heart attacks. Most people can increase their MET capacity by 10 to 20 percent within three months of starting an exercise program.

physiologist Bob Greene (Oprah Winfrey's personal trainer) to promote the health benefits of walking—and, not coincidentally, a new product called the Go Active! Happy Meal. It was a step in the right direction, particularly from a company that isn't exactly synonymous with healthy eating. The promotion ultimately fizzled because consumers didn't line up to buy the leaner Happy Meal. But the science behind the promotion was solid.

Walking is the ideal exercise. Most of us will never be world-class athletes. And few people care for heart rates, optimal training schedules, or weight-lifting and aerobic workouts. We just want to lose weight, feel stronger, be healthier, and get a little extra energy in the bargain. Walking gives you all of this without your ever having to break a sweat.

Greene's approach was simplicity itself: take at least 10,000 steps a day. That's it. No heart monitors, no gym memberships, no trendy exercise outfits. Just put one foot in front of the other 10,000 times. If you do this, and also trim about 250 to 500 calories a day from your current diet, you'll easily lose the 10 percent of your body weight that doctors say will *significantly* reduce your risk of serious disease and help you live longer. Folks, it doesn't get any simpler than that.

This isn't about fitness; it's about *fatness*. And fatness is what's killing us, not un-fitness. A recent study by Johns Hopkins Medical School confirms that being overweight is a bigger risk factor for cardiovascular disease than being unfit. Losing weight, the doctors concluded, is more important than getting fit when it comes to avoiding a heart attack.

Now, 10,000 steps may sound like a lot, but it's really not. Confirmed couch potatoes already take about 2,000 to 3,000 steps a day. So even if you were a sedentary slug (which I'm sure you're not), you're already one-third of the way there. With just a little extra effort, 10,000 daily steps (the equivalent of four to five miles a day) is a piece of cake. Add this to the small, painless diet changes you've just learned about, and not only will you stop gaining weight, but you can easily drop two pounds (or more) a week. That's *every* week. You do the math: You'll be 8 pounds lighter in a month . . . shed 24 pounds in three months . . . drop almost 50 pounds in six months . . . and be 100 pounds lighter than your current weight just one year after you say, "I'll do it!"

That's without subsisting on tofu and sprouts. Or giving up fast food. Or joining a gym. Or popping dangerous, expensive pills. Or any of that other silliness that just doesn't work.

This diet plan does work because it fits so neatly into your normal life—and because it's not asking you to deprive yourself of any of life's pleasures.

The Easiest Calorie-Burner Ever

Walking is something you can do without lessons or specialized gear. You don't need to be in great shape to start. All you have to do is lace up your walking shoes and go. The very simplicity of walking may have worked against its reputation as a weight-loss tool. It seems too easy to be effective. But consider this: A study at Texas Woman's University found that people who walked at a moderate pace three miles a day (about 6,000 steps), five days a week, achieved the same cardiovascular benefits as joggers. And brisk walking can actually burn *more* calories than jogging!

Start walking today and you'll start losing weight almost immediately. And, as with compound interest at the bank, the results will multiply the longer you do it. That's because physical activity not only burns calories immediately, it also keeps your metabolism revved up, so your body continues to burn extra calories while you're watching *Desperate Housewives* or *Monday Night Football*—or sleeping in your bed. Walking also builds muscle; and muscle burns seventy times more calories than fat.

I don't believe in hard-core workouts for nonathletes because I've seen too many people hurt themselves—and that's not the worst of it. Average people who exercise too hard are at risk for permanent joint damage, stroke, and heart attack. Mild exercise, on the other hand, imposes none of these risks. Going for a walk, even if you walk slowly, promotes lower blood pressure, better circulation, and healthier cholesterol profiles. Walking makes the body's cells more responsive to insulin and improves their ability to remove glucose from the blood. It also lowers blood sugar by burning glucose for fuel. Best of all, it promotes weight loss—especially from the tummy—which further lowers diabetes risk.

The landmark Diabetes Prevention Program study found that walking daily for thirty minutes at a moderate pace, along with the simple, painless diet changes I've already outlined, can reduce your risk of developing diabetes by 58 percent. If you already have the condition, walking will slow the progression of the disease and lower your chances of blindness or limb amputation.

The fitness fanatics have it all wrong. The fact is, exercise is a rather *poor* way to lose weight. To lose one pound of fat through exercise alone, a person needs to burn 3,500 calories in addition to what they're currently burning. For a 170-pound person to lose 2 pounds a week without dietary changes, he or she would have to walk at least ten miles a day. It takes an hour on a treadmill to work off the calories from one medium-size bagel—and that's without butter or cream cheese!

The Fast-Food Diet Plan is a much easier way to go. To lose one pound a week, you need a calorie *deficit* of 500 daily calories. (Double that if you want to lose two pounds per week.) The most painless way to achieve this deficit is to hit the calorie equation from both sides: Consume fewer calories every day and burn off a few extra ones. You don't have to eat any less; just eat smarter. Hold the cheese on a burger. Don't go for the special sauce on a Big Mac. Substitute seltzer water for one of your daily soft drinks. These three tiny sacrifices in one day could save you those 500 calories. Go for a walk at lunchtime or after dinner, and you've achieved your 1,000 calorie savings for the day! Want to lose more and lose faster? No problem. It's all up to you.

Once you get the hang of how easy this strategy is, you'll

find yourself making these smart little shifts throughout your entire day. You'll be able to cut 1,000 calories from your daily diet and never even miss them. But here's the best part. As soon as you begin to see the results on your bathroom scale, in your bedroom mirror, and in how loose your clothes start to fit, you'll be "bitten by the bug." *Your weight loss will naturally accelerate because there's no better motivation than success.* As you actually experience how this "brainpower strategy" really delivers results, there will be no stopping you.

Count Your Steps, Lose Your Pounds

So how can you tell if you're taking 10,000 steps a day? The easiest way is to buy a good pedometer and hang it on your belt or shoe. This clever device counts each step you take and gives you the total whenever you want to know. You can launch into a calorie-burning walking program without any gadgetry at all, but pedometers are a great way to figure out where you're starting from and how much farther you need to go. (If you can't find a good pedometer, check our free Web site at www.thefastfooddiet.com for some suggestions from top-of-the-line models to cheapies that are quite serviceable.)

As I mentioned, people who are relatively sedentary take 2,000 to 3,000 steps a day. If that's you, it's not going to feel so good to jump to 10,000 steps right away. And if something doesn't feel good, most folks aren't going to stay with it. So I've devised a smarter approach. Going from zero to 60 right away, so to speak, could be too much for your regular routine—as well as for your muscles. You don't have to think of 10,000 steps as a "rule" or some magic number. Your body will start losing weight below that amount. There's no need to rush. Give yourself time to get your muscles and cardiovascular system into shape. This transition happens more quickly than you might think. When it does, increase the number of daily steps *gradually*. That's the key phrase to remember. Easy does it every time. When your added activity begins to feel easy, increase it again. Keep going until you hit 10,000 steps. At that point, you can keep adding, or walk more quickly to get your heart and lungs pumping. That's when the pounds really start melting away.

This 10,000-step approach is equivalent to the amount of daily activity recommended by the surgeon general to reduce the size of your waistline and your risk of serious disease. Once you've clipped a pedometer to your belt, you can keep track of how many steps you normally take just while going about your business: walking to the mailbox, going up and down stairs, moving the hose in the yard, and so on. All of these steps add up. Research shows that it's the *total* amount of activity you get in a day that makes a difference. The pounds will drop away whether you take those steps all at once or incrementally throughout the day.

Most people clip on their pedometer first thing in the morning so it will record their steps all day. Or you can use a pedometer just when you're walking. There are a few types of pedometers:

- **Counting pedometers**   These are the simplest and least expensive. They count the steps you take, and the display shows either the number of steps, the distance you've covered, or both.

- **Walking speedometers and odometers**   These are a little fancier. Some include displays that count steps, but they're used mainly to track your speed and distance.

- **Multifunction pedometers**   If you're one of those people who love data, these models are for you. They can be set to display the steps you've taken, the calories you've burned, the speed you're going, and how far you've traveled. Some models also have stopwatches, pulse readers, and seven-day memories. Would you like your pedometer to talk to you and monitor your progress with a global positioning system (GPS)? You can get those, too.

Once the pedometer is up and running (the instructions tell you how to adjust it to your normal walking stride), you can start counting steps and decide how far (or how fast) you'll want to go. Remember, you don't have to take all your steps at one time. You're already walking throughout the day. Those steps count toward the total. Get a sense of what you're currently doing, and then add from there. Here are some other helpful tips.

Establish your baseline   Put on your pedometer first thing in the morning. Wear it all day, and chart how many steps you're currently taking. That's your baseline level. You might find, for example, that walking to a nearby convenience store to fetch the newspaper adds up to 1,200 steps. Walking to a neighbor's might add up to 800 steps. And taking your dog around the park might give you another 1,000 to 2,000 steps. Steps, like calories, add up quickly.

Kick it up 10 percent   After you've established your basic walking routine for a week, you may want to boost your average daily steps by 10 percent. If your baseline was, say, 4,000 steps a day, try to increase it consistently by 400 steps a day. It doesn't take more than a few minutes to walk 400 steps—and remember, you don't have to do it all at once. Your intent is to increase your daily average. So you might take one extra turn around the block, or find an excuse to go up and down the stairs once or twice, or ditch the remote control and change the channels by hand. *Every step counts!* Stay at this baseline-plus-10-percent level for a few

Your Success Is a Shoe-in

Your feet absorb the equivalent of about double your body weight with each step you take. Good shoes are critical for comfort and to prevent injury. Plan on spending at least $65 for walking or running shoes with a low heel and cushioned, flexible sole.

While you're at the store, check out the athletic socks made of synthetic material, such as Sorbtek. They have cushioning in the heel and ball of the foot, and fabrics that draw perspiration away from the skin to keep your feet dry and free of blisters.

Don't let winter's blustery chill keep you inside and off your feet. Dress in layers: a light jacket over a sweatshirt over a T-shirt. You can bundle up when you're chilled, and remove a layer or two once you heat up. Also, wear a hat to minimize heat loss. In cold weather, anywhere from 20 to 60 percent of heat is lost through the scalp.

Remember to wear white or reflective clothing for safety. You can buy reflective vests at sporting goods stores for about $15.

days or a few weeks—however long it takes for it to seem easy. When it does, kick it up another 10 percent. Your body's "pleasure principle" will let you know if you're overdoing it.

Keep a log   At the end of each day, jot down how many steps you took and how far you walked. Better yet, write down how many steps it took to reach specific destinations—say, 1,200 steps to the convenience store . . . 1,000 steps to walk around the park . . . and so on. You don't have to keep a log indefinitely, but it's a good way to get a sense of which activities add significant numbers of steps to your day.

Kick it up a notch   You don't have to go all-out when you're working toward the 10,000-step goal. Even once you've reached it, you might decide you prefer to walk leisurely. Every walk, even a slow stroll, will burn calories and boost your cardiovascular fitness. But you'll burn more calories if you step a little faster. Suppose you walk at a brisk clip of four miles an hour. Your diet stays the same, and you do all of your serious walking in one sixty-minute stretch. Just walking like this four days a week for a year (with no diet changes at all) will knock 18 pounds off your frame. I'd say that qualifies as serious success.

A Week-by-Week Walking Plan

Exercise scientists are fond of issuing weight-loss prescriptions that are so difficult and time-consuming that no reasonable person follows them in real life. Why make things difficult? Studies clearly show that thirty minutes of daily exercise provides all the health and fitness benefits most people need and desire.

Walking is easy; the hard part is to stay with it. More than 50 percent of adults who start a fitness program give it up within a year—and most quit sooner than that. Why? Because we humans are creatures of habit. Scientists have found that it takes us about twenty-eight days to break an old habit and establish a new one. (That's why most drug and alcohol rehab programs are twenty-eight days long.) So being consistent in the beginning is important. Skipping a few days of walking just makes it harder to lock this new programming into place.

The famously successful Twelve-Step program works because it tackles the problem of breaking old habits and establishing new ones one day at a time. I suggest you approach your weight-loss goals the same way. Don't think about losing 100 pounds (that's why people fail; the task is too big)—instead, think about the small steps you'll take today. To help you, I've organized my walking program into a week-by-week plan. Please don't feel bound to it, or you'll rebel against it. Think of it as a kind of map to your final destination.

Week 1   Consider this your break-in period. It's not important how many steps you take or what you see on the bathroom scale. All that's important is getting your feet moving—and wearing the pedometer all day so you can keep track. Go about your usual routine. Try to add steps, but don't worry about it. Just seeing the pedometer will keep the idea of walking firmly in your mind. You'll probably take extra steps just because you're thinking about it.

- Each morning, reset the pedometer. Wear it all day, except when you're in the shower.

- At night, remove the pedometer and write down how many steps you took. If you did anything unusual during the day that added or subtracted steps—for example, you logged a lot of extra steps at the mall, or it rained and you didn't walk the dog—write that down, too.

- At the end of the week, figure out the average number of steps you took each day. This is your starting place, or baseline.

Week 2   By now, your body is warming up to exercise. Start pushing yourself—not hard, just enough so that you're taking more average daily steps than you did the first week. Notice that progress feels good. You're gaining personal power.

- Increase your average daily steps by 10 percent. If you took an average of 4,000 steps a day during the first week, increase it to 4,400 steps. Some days you'll do more, and some days you'll do less. Think about averages rather than absolute numbers.

■ Look for excuses to increase your average. When you're talking on the phone, stand up and walk in place. You'll be amazed how the steps add up during even a brief conversation. You might find yourself thinking, "I just had a 220-step conversation." Take the stairs instead of elevators. Park at the back of parking lots so you take an extra few hundred steps going to and from the car.

■ At the end of the week, calculate the average number of steps you took each day.

Week 3   You'll *know* you're getting in better shape at this point. You'll feel extra strength and energy in your body—and you should start seeing the benefits on the scale. Just as important as the immediate gain is the fact that walking might start to feel pleasurable—something you *want* to do, rather than have to do.

■ If you're not yet averaging 10,000 daily steps, increase your daily total by another 10 percent. If you were taking 4,400 steps the previous week, increase it to 4,800 this week—or however much feels right to you.

■ If you're the type that likes an extra challenge, increase the intensity of the walking (by going faster) or the distance (by taking extra steps). In addition, incorporate a minute or two of stretching into your routine. About five minutes into a walk, for example, lean down and grip your ankles, keeping your knees together. Or take a big step forward with one leg, bend the knee, and stretch until your thigh is parallel to the ground. Stretching after you've warmed up with a short walk is a great way to stay limber and prevent injuries. Besides, the extra exertion burns extra calories.

- Bend your arms at the elbows and pump them as you walk. It increases stress on the cardiovascular system and also allows you to move faster. Hint: You're walking too fast if you're too out of breath to talk as you walk.

Week 4   You can actually feel that your heart and lungs are in much better shape. You're noticeably thinner. And your muscles are primed for more (and faster) walking.

- Keep pushing toward the 10,000-step goal. If you're already there, keep going! If not, increase your steps, again, by about 10 percent, or whichever amount feels comfortable.

- Get in the habit of checking the pedometer a few times a day to see how you're progressing. If the day's half done, and you haven't come close to your halfway step point, you'll need to get your feet moving. Try not to let yourself fall short. Find reasons to walk more, even if that means just spending more of the day standing and moving your feet, instead of sitting.

- Want more challenge? Push your speed a little further. If you walk as fast as you would if you were late for an appointment, and maintain that pace for five or ten minutes, your heart will be beating at between 65 and 85 percent of its maximum rate. This is the so-called target zone, at which point your body is burning calories at its most efficient rate. Note: If you want to exercise in your target zone, I suggest you first get permission from your doctor. Some of you may need an exercise stress test to help screen you for hidden heart disease.

- Bunch your hands into fists when you walk and pump your arms. This improves your aerodynamics and increases your comfortable speed.

Week 5 and beyond   By now, you're strong enough to increase your walking distances, and your cardiovascular system is up to a faster pace. You may even feel like taking a longer hike in the woods on weekends. Moving your body definitely feels good by now. You're in the groove, which means that logging a lot of daily steps feels better than sitting on your rump. Exercise, in other words, is becoming a habit. Congratulations!

At this point in the program, you probably have a pretty good idea of how many steps you're taking in a certain amount of time. You might decide to continue using the pedometer and keeping the daily logs, but you don't have to. As long as you keep moving toward (or beyond) 10,000 daily steps—and also experiment with your walking speed by, for example, walking fast for 500 to 1,000 steps, slowing down for 500 steps, and then increasing the speed again—you're probably losing anywhere from half a pound to one pound a week. Remember, that's without factoring in any of your eating changes.

Some people will really be feeling their oats by now and will enjoy the challenge of pushing themselves a bit more. If that's you, try this:

■ As you walk, contract your abdominal muscles for four to ten seconds, or until the muscles fatigue. Relax and walk normally for a few minutes, then repeat the contractions.

■ Plan your walks so that you encounter a hill or flight of stairs after about five minutes. As you climb, briefly squeeze the quadriceps, the muscle in the front of the upper thigh, as your foot hits the ground. Alternate legs as you go.

■ Work your arms by pumping them while you walk.

Dealing with Boredom

If you stick with this 10,000-step plan, you're guaranteed to be stronger and fitter. How much weight you lose is really up to you. If you walk s-l-o-w-l-y, you'll burn calories, but not enough to immediately see the results on the scale. A leisurely ten-minute walk burns only 3 to 4 calories a minute—not very practical when you realize that you have to burn 3,500 calories to lose a pound of fat. For serious weight loss, you'll want to increase the effort and walk faster or longer—or both.

"You mean I have to *keep* doing this?" some patients ask me. Well, yes. Short-term efforts give only short-term results.

Leash and Lose

By some estimates, about as many American dogs as American owners are overweight. If your dog looks as though he's gobbled too many biscuits, do both of you a favor by hooking up a leash and heading outside. A new study reports that people who walk a dog can lose substantial amounts of weight.

During the fifty-week study, people initially walked "loaner" dogs for ten minutes a day, three times a week. They worked up to twenty-minute walks, five days a week. After fifty weeks, the dog-walkers lost an average of 14 pounds. That's a better result than most people achieve with conventional weight-loss plans.

The study also looked at people who followed the same dog-walking plan for only twenty-six weeks. They lost weight, but not as much as the long-timers. If you own a dog, of course, you're already in it for the long haul. So make the commitment and walk. You can always make an exception on rainy days. They're a good excuse to watch *Lassie* reruns.

That's what dieting is all about—and why its results are temporary. We're talking about your life, not your college reunion. It doesn't matter how much weight you lose this month if you gain it all back later.

Boredom is a weight-loss killer. All of us, including serious athletes, get bored with our routines. People who are new to exercise tend to feel bored more quickly because they don't have a strong, positive habit yet. The secret to long-term success is to build variation into your routine so it stays mentally and physically challenging. Losing weight is a powerful motivator in itself, but psychologists have found that you'll need more than that if you hope to succeed long-term. Here's what they recommend:

Up the challenge   Turn your walks into workouts by changing *how* you walk. Walking with extra weight, for example, boosts cardiovascular exertion. You can buy vests at sporting goods stores that have pockets for inserting small weights. This way the load is distributed evenly over the body. Avoid ankle or wrist weights, as well as carrying hand weights. They concentrate the load in one small area and increase the risk of joint injury.

Walk and lunge   This is too strenuous to do in the first month of your workout, but walking lunges are a superb way to increase metabolism by strengthening the large muscles in the thighs. Walk as you normally do for five or ten minutes. Then take a long, lunging step with your right foot, lowering your right thigh until it's parallel to the ground (the left knee will almost touch the ground). Hold for a second, then rise and pull forward, lunging forward with your left leg. Repeat eight to ten times with both legs, then start walking normally again. These "walking lunges" develop strength and flexibility in the lower body. At the same time, working these large muscles increases the amount of oxygen the body uses. People with high oxygen use have fewer heart attacks and live longer than those with lower oxygen use.

Hit the hills   To stay challenged throughout your program, look for harder places to walk: steep streets, mountain trails, or multiple flights of stairs are all good choices. You don't have to be a speed demon. Just put more stress on your legs and heart and lungs.

Raise the bar   Maybe you walk 10,000 steps most days of the week. Set aside a few days to bump up the amount—say, to 12,000 or even 14,000 steps. If you go all in one shot, which would probably take about forty-five minutes, your metabolism will be buzzing like a hummingbird's. Weight falls off quickly when exercise intensity increases.

Join the crowds   People who start a walking program tend to stick with it longer when they do it with others. Face it, it can get lonely out there by yourself. It's more fun to walk with a buddy or a bunch. Look into 5K or 10K walk/run events—or charity walks. You'll meet a lot of like-minded people—and you might hook up with a regular walking partner.

Get some baseline measurements   It's easy to see progress in other people, but not so easy to notice it in yourself. Apart from taking before-and-after pictures or keeping close tabs on the bathroom scale, you might want to ask your doctor to measure your body mass index (BMI) and establish baseline measurements for cholesterol and blood pressure. Every one of these signposts should improve, sometimes dramatically, within a few months. That kind of feedback—knowing you've lost, say, 5 percent of your body fat, and dropped your blood pressure a few points—gives you powerful motivation to keep going.

Take advantage of TV time   The great thing about the 10,000-step program is that you don't have to set aside time just for walking. Yes, regular activity is ideal for weight loss, but every step counts. So don't just take up couch space while you're watching TV. Stand up and walk in place. Do it for just one sitcom (including commercials), and you'll come close to hitting your 10,000 steps right there.

Stay positive   Everyone goes through periods when progress seems to grind to a halt. Maybe you've been walking for three or four months. The first few months, the pounds just seemed to drop by themselves. But lately, the scale hardly budges, and you're getting tired of all the work—and you're *still* heavier than you'd like to be. It's easy at this point to start losing steam. Nip this negative thinking pattern in the bud by focusing on your progress! This is the time to remind yourself of how far you've come, not how far you've got to go. Nothing short-circuits motivation faster than focusing on the future. Focus instead on the weight you have lost. Find encouragement in each small victory, even if that's only a quarter or half a pound. Those small amounts add up, and if you keep walking, it's unlikely they'll ever come back.

CHAPTER 15

The Future of Fast Food

You'd think from recent headlines that the fast-food giants are facing a soul-searching crisis in the face of lawsuits and demands from consumers to serve healthier food. Not quite. True, the chains have bowed (somewhat) to nutritional critics. They are afraid of being sued, as tobacco companies were, for putting ingredients *known* to cause health problems in the public's food supply. McDonald's, for example, recently pledged to stop cooking its french fries in trans-fat oil. Arby's has introduced a new line of Market Fresh sandwiches. But it's naive to think that large-scale changes are coming any time soon. This is a $110 *billion* industry built on food that's high in fat, high in calories, and dished out in super-large sizes. This is what customers still line up for.

But things are changing—and the push is coming from consumers who want healthier, leaner food. Right now, about 75 percent of all restaurant meals in North America are fast food.

Consumers aren't going to quit McDonald's or Burger King or Wendy's. But they are beginning to request more healthful options. And don't think the mega-chains aren't noticing. These are savvy businesspeople who make their money by giving the public what they want. More and more people are starting to make the connection between what they eat and how they look, feel, and live.

Doubt it? Do you realize that Americans already spend upward of $32 billion annually on all types of natural and organic products? Nearly half of U.S. consumers say they use organic products at least occasionally. And organic food is now a $15-billion-a-year business, growing 20 percent a year. It's no exaggeration to say that North Americans are more concerned with good nutrition, health, and weight loss than ever before. They want healthier food and they are voting with their dollars and charge cards. If the big chains don't provide what they're looking for, they'll go to places that will.

I know healthy fast food sounds like an oxymoron, but there's no reason fast food can't taste good and be nutritious at the same time. In the last couple of years, a few daring new entrepreneurs have started to provide just that: fast food that is slimming and healthful. Some examples:

O'Naturals   This small, Maine-based fast-food chain has a handful of franchises serving all-natural, organic foods, with a large selection of vegetarian, low-fat, and low-calorie entrée items. Founder Gary Hirshberg, who also launched the Stonyfield Farm yogurt company, hopes to expand the chain to include more than a hundred restaurants within ten years.

Healthy Bites Grill   Another promising new contender for the nation's fast-food dollars. With just a few outlets, the Florida-based company doesn't even qualify as an annoyance to the big chains. But with veggie and buffalo burgers, baked fries, and a juice bar, it's well-positioned to expand its operation by catering to consumers who are interested more in *fresh* and *healthy* than in merely *big*.

Topz   They advertise the "leanest burgers in America," and now have more than half a dozen restaurants in California, Michigan, and Texas. Founder Mark Avila, a lifelong burger lover, decided to create a cheeseburger with 50 percent less fat than his competitors. The average fast-food burger has some 35 grams of fat. At Topz, a fully loaded one has 15 grams.

Zone Café   My favorite, not just because I joined with Dr. Barry Sears (founder of the Zone Diet programs) in developing this chain of fast-food restaurants. I love the Zone Café because it features some of the healthiest food available ("fast" or otherwise), such as Alaskan salmon (mercury-free), turkey wraps, veggie salads, hormone-and-antibiotic-free organic bison burgers, and a variety of foods rich in omega-3 fatty acids, such as broiled tuna. Menu items have detailed nutritional information. When you receive your cash register receipt, it also shows you the total of calories, carbs, and fat you consumed. In the next year, we expect to have restaurants throughout Connecticut, Florida, Arizona, and Nevada—with many more to come.

Subway   They really started it all. While Subway doesn't promote itself as a "natural" chain, it could do so. It is unique among the big fast-food chains in that it offers more than a token number of low-fat, low-calorie choices. If you order a sub on a whole-grain roll, pile it with vegetables, and hold the mayo, you'll be getting one of the healthiest meals you can eat away from home. With nearly 25,000 restaurants in eighty-one countries, Subway has proved that "fresh and healthy" sells.

The Weight-Loss Future

This is no temporary health fad; it is a healthy trend: tomorrow's fast-food joints will be filled with menu items that clean your arteries, regulate your blood sugar, control your waistline, give you plenty of energy to burn—and still taste yummy. The day is coming when every restaurant, from the sit-down and fast-food chains to the corner pizzeria, will offer consumers a good selection of entrées made only with healthy fats, low-glycemic carbohydrates, and an abundance of garden-fresh fruits and vegetables. None of us is likely to eat healthy all the time, but most of us would like to do it *more* of the time. When you consider that the average North American eats outside the home at least three times a week, the change to healthier ingredients in restaurants will make it far easier for everyone to whittle away at those stubborn pounds, while at the same time reducing the nutritional risk factors that contribute to today's serious chronic diseases.

A few years ago, I would have called this a fantasy. Today, it's already beginning to happen. Thanks to pressure from consumers, as well as from the new "healthful" chains, the fast-food kings are taking baby steps in the right direction. No longer must you choose between ordering the salad (and leaving hungry) and wolfing down a cheeseburger and supersized fries. If you're eating light, you can choose among items like a fruit cup, a lean chicken breast, and grilled salmon, depending on the chain. You can order a large, unsweetened iced tea instead of the usual soft drink. Fruit juices, whole-grain rolls, tuna or whole-grain salads—the choice is yours. Of course, you can still have the grease-burger and fries when you're in the mood. But you aren't locked into anything, and you definitely aren't stuck with a pallid bowl of iceberg lettuce.

As a cardiologist, I'd be thrilled if every person in this country would eat a healthier diet. Sure, I'd have fewer patients, but that would be just fine with me. Good doctors are happy when people are healthier. With restaurants like Topz and Zone Café leading the way, it's going to happen. At these and other healthy chains, consumers don't have to hunt and peck through the menu to find something that's remotely healthy—or at least only moderately bad. Almost anything they order is going to be suitably lean and nutritious.

The Zone Café shows how easy this can be. Every item on the menu is something you might see in a restaurant while strolling down a cobblestone street in Italy or along the beach in Greece. The ingredients are fresh and natural, free of harmful chemicals and antibiotics. The carbohydrates are all low-glycemic: They're digested slowly in the intestine and only gradually release their glucose payload. This is what prevents those sudden insulin surges that make calories much more likely to be stored as fat. The lean protein on the menu is optimal for controlling appetite. Enormous portions simply aren't necessary, because the foods are naturally filling. And finally, the menu includes a lot of foods that are high in omega-3 fatty acids, anti-inflammatory substances that greatly reduce the risk of disease.

What you won't find at Zone Café or similar restaurants are the usual saturated and trans fats. Both of these fats, which are used by the bucketful at the big chains, have been linked to stroke, high blood pressure, heart disease, and some cancers. Scientists have found that saturated fat in the diet generates enormous amounts of free radicals, those toxic molecules that trigger inflammation that damages cells throughout the body, including in the heart and arteries, and possibly in the brain as well. The darned thing is, food doesn't need *any* of these fats to be delicious.

If you order the Wild Alaskan Salmon Burger at Zone Café, you'll get healthy amounts of omega-3 fatty acids. Along with olive oil, these fats are so beneficial. The omega-3s and olive oil have anti-inflammatory properties, which greatly reduce the risk of cardiovascular disease—by close to 30 percent, in some cases. They also play a role in lowering blood pressure, controlling cholesterol, and reducing the risk of blood-stopping clots in the arteries.

Since the salmon is accompanied by generous servings of spring greens and fresh vegetables, you'll get the benefit of strongly protective antioxidants, along with healthy amounts of fiber. Thanks to the fiber, low-glycemic carbohydrates, healthy fats, and lean protein, you could eat out like this every day and almost be sure of losing weight.

I'm using the Zone Café as an example because it's a project close to my heart. But you can find nearly all of the same benefits at many of the new, healthier chains.

The Ahi Fillet Burger at Topz, for example, has all of the healthy fats that you'd expect to get from fish, with only 2 grams of saturated fat and 360 calories. Want a drink with that? Forget the usual sugar- and calorie-loaded soft drinks. At Topz, you can order a fruit-filled shake (peach, raspberry, and more) with barely 200 calories and very little saturated fat. All that fruit will flood your body with natural nutritional substances that are particularly good for you.

The Veggie Garden Grill at Evos (a small, Florida-based fast-food restaurant), with only 310 calories and no saturated fat, is as lean as it could possibly be. Yet because the vegetables are grilled, they're sweet and smoky and rich-tasting—the opposite of bland. Want to feed your meat tooth? Try the Santa

Fe Adobo Turkey. It has hardly any more calories than the veggie grill, and only 1 gram of saturated fat. Crispy Thai Trout, Honey Mesquite Chicken, Evos Free-range Steakburger—with menu entrées like these, you'd think you're eating at a high-end restaurant instead of a fast-food chain. It's amazing what's already possible!

These new healthful fast-food chains are still in their early days, so you might not find one in your neighborhood just yet. But they're coming, and their example is inspiring. Even if you continue to eat at traditional fast-food or sit-down restaurants once a week or so, you can still control your weight and eat better by ordering a little more thoughtfully—by listening to your waistline, following your taste buds, and heeding some of the tips in this book.

As mentioned early on, get in the habit of ordering chicken that's grilled instead of fried—and having it more often than beef. Applebee's offers a Sizzling Chicken Skillet that has only 360 calories and 4 grams of fat. Have a taste for something closer to traditional junk food? A Thin 'N Crispy at Pizza Hut, topped with olives, mushrooms, and other vegetables, has less than 4 grams of saturated fat and under 200 calories. Pizza as a weight-loss tool? It sure *can* be.

With the thousands of weight-loss books that have been published in the last ten years, and the billions of dollars spent on weight-loss clinics, programs, and seminars, you'd think that we'd have it all figured out by now. Unfortunately, what you often get are gimmicks—or just as bad, unrealistic prescriptions that have no bearing on how most of us actually live.

The Fast-Food Diet is hardly a prescription to eat fast food at every meal. I certainly don't advocate eating the majority of your meals away from home. If you do that consistently, losing weight can be a real battle. What *The Fast-Food Diet* shows you is how to eat smarter at fast-food and sit-down restaurants—and how to incorporate some of the principles of healthier cooking at home.

People in Asia and the Mediterranean countries tend to stay lean and healthy because they consistently eat fresher food, more produce, less meat and saturated fat, and fewer sugary items. They load up on whole grains, beans, and fruit and veggies—foods that are filling with a minimum of calories. They also drink moderate amounts of red wine or green tea and walk or bicycle far more than we do. Those are the goals we should be shooting for, because hundreds of scientific studies prove that they prevent disease, keep you slim and healthy, and increase your life span.

If you now eat the typical American diet, you're not going to achieve this overnight. But a good place to start is by making smarter picks when you dine out. You don't have to completely overhaul your lifestyle or force yourself to eat foods that you really don't like. The solution is in making small, painless shifts *right now*. Like a snowball rolling down a hill, these tiny changes will gain a momentum of their own—and they'll add up to big improvements in your weight, your health, your self-confidence, and your happiness.

Think about that the next time you're heading out for lunch.

APPENDIX A

The Glycemic Foods Index

Low-Glycemic-Index Foods (GI < 55):
Low Inducers of Insulin

Stone-ground whole-wheat bread	53	Apple juice (fresh in season)	40
Sourdough bread	52	Plums	39
Kiwis	52	Meat ravioli	39
Kellogg's All-Bran with extra fiber	51	Pears	38
		Apples	38
Pumpernickel bread	51	Flavored low-fat yogurt	33
Very dark chocolate	49	Chickpeas	33
Oatmeal	49	Skim milk	32
Green peas	48	Egg fettuccine	32
Baked beans	48	Dried apricots	31
Orange juice (fresh)	46	Lentils	30
Grapes	46	Whole milk	27
Kellogg's Bran Buds with psyllium	45	Kidney beans	27
		Cherries	22
Oranges	44	Peanuts	14

Moderate-Glycemic-Index Foods (GI 55 to 70):
Moderate Inducers of Insulin

White bread	70	Shortbread	64
Whole-wheat bread	69	Beets*	64
Post Shredded Wheat	67	New potatoes*	62
Cantaloupes*	65	Ice cream	61
Sucrose	65	Long-grain white rice	56
Raisins*	64	Brown rice	55

High-Glycemic-Index Foods (GI > 70):
Rapid Inducers of Insulin

Glucose	100	Waffles	76
Baked potatoes*	93	French fries	75
Red-skinned potatoes*	88	Graham crackers	75
Kellogg's Corn Flakes	84	Kellogg's Raisin Bran	73
Pretzels	83	Short-grain white rice	72
Kellogg's Rice Krispies	82	Bagels	72
Jelly beans	80	Watermelon*	72
Vanilla wafers	77	Corn chips	72
Rye bread	76		

*These foods have other benefits, such as a high antioxidant level. Don't avoid them just because of the glycemic index value.

APPENDIX B

Low-Calorie Snacks

Snacking is essential if you want to lose weight, because it keeps your hunger under control. Ideally, you want to eat something every three hours so you don't become ravenous and eat everything in sight at your next meal. The ideal snack should contain no more than 250 calories—and those calories should not be from refined carbohydrates, otherwise your blood sugar will spike and then drop, triggering more hunger. As with everything you eat, your snack should have a little protein and fat in it. This way it will satisfy you longer. Here's a list of my favorite snacks. Feel free to add your own as long as you follow my "healthy snack" guidelines.

Source	Food	Calories	Fat (grams)
Convenience store	Stonyfield's Organic Smoothie Style Yogurt (small container)	150	2
	Stonyfield's Organic Low-fat Yogurt (small container)	140	1.5
	Part-skim mozzarella cheese stick	70	4
	Swiss Amish Cheese (1 oz.)	91	6
	with apple (1)	163	6
	Macadamia nuts or walnuts (1/2 oz.)	110	11

Source	Food	Calories	Fat (grams)
Home	Apple or pear	72–81	0
	with mixed nuts (1 tbsp.)	197	14
	Homemade granola with nuts (1 handful)	150	8
	Grapes (one bunch)	110	0
	Blueberries or raspberries (1 handful)	105	0
	Banana (1)	105	0
	Walnuts (1 handful)	175	17
	Celery stick (1) and hard-boiled egg (1) (remove yellow center [yolk] and fill w/hummus)	105	8
Vending Machine	Mixed dried fruit & nuts	160–180	8
	Roasted peanuts/almonds (1 oz.)	160	14
	Nuts/trail mix (small bag) (1½ oz.)	230	12
Health Food Store	Power Bar	240	3
	Balance Bar	200	6
	Think Organic Fruit and Nut Snack Bar	190	9
	Kelp Krunch	130	8
Supermarket	Trail mix (1 oz.)	194	12
	Almonds (1 handful)	207	18
Panera Bread	Half blueberry bagel with low-fat cream cheese	290	4.5
Dunkin' Donuts	Half multigrain bagel with 1 tbsp. low-fat cream cheese	225	5
Auntie Anne's	Half Garlic Pretzel (dry: no butter or topping)	160	1
TCBY	Tropical Replenisher Smoothie	240	0
McDonald's	Fruit 'n Yogurt Parfait	160	2
Orange Julius	Muscle Peach Smoothie (20 oz.)	260	0.5
	Orange Original (16 oz.)	220	1

For a more complete listing of low-calorie weight-loss snacks, go to our free Web site at www.thefastfooddiet.com.

Bibliography

Astrup A. "Super-sized and diabetic by frequent fast-food consumption?" *Lancet* 2005;365:4–5.

Barnard, Neal. *Breaking the Food Seduction: The Hidden Reasons Behind Food Cravings—and 7 Steps to End Them Naturally.* New York: St. Martin's Press, 2003.

———. *Turn Off the Fat Genes: The Revolutionary Guide to Losing Weight.* New York: Harmony Books, 2001.

Bes-Rastrollo M, Sánchez-Villegas A, Gómez-Garcia E, Martinez JA, Pajares RM, Martinez-González MA. "Predictors of weight gain in a Mediterranean cohort: the Seguimiento Universidad de Navarra Study." *Am J Clin Nutr* 1983;2:362–70.

Brand-Miller JC. "Glycemic load and chronic disease." *Nutr Rev* 2003;61:S49–55.

Bray GA, Nielsen SJ, Opokin BM. "Consumption of high-fructose corn syrup in beverages may play a role in the epidemic of obesity." *Am J Clin Nutr* 2004;79:537–43.

Brownell, Kelly D., and Katherine Battle Horgen. *Food Fight: The Inside Story of the Food Industry, America's Obesity Crisis, and What We Can Do about It.* New York: McGraw-Hill, 2004.

Burani, Johanna, and Lina Rao. *Good Carbs, Bad Carbs: An Indispensable Guide to Eating the Right Carbs for Losing Weight and Optimum Health.* New York: Marlowe & Company, 2002.

Campbell, T. Colin, and Thomas M. Campbell II. *The China Study: Startling Implications for Diet, Weight Loss and Long-term Health.* Dallas, Tex: BenBella Books, 2004.

225

Coulston AM, Hollenbeck CB, Swislocki AL, Reaven GM. "Effect of source of dietary carbohydrate on plasma glucose and insulin responses to mixed meals in subjects with NIDDM." *Diabetes Care* 1987;10:395–400.

Ebbeling CB, Sinclair KB, Pereira MA, Garcia-Lago E, Feldman HA, Ludwig DS. "Compensation of energy intake from fast food among overweight and lean adolescents." *JAMA* 2004;291: 2828–33.

Elliott SS, Keim NL, Stern JS, Teff K, Harvel PJ. "Fructose, weight gain, and the insulin resistance syndrome." *Am J Clin Nutr* 2002;76:911–22.

Lisle, Douglas J., and Alan Goldhamer. *The Pleasure Trap: Mastering the Hidden Force That Undermines Health and Happiness.* Summertown, Tenn.: Healthy Living Publications, an imprint of Book Publishing Company, 2003.

Ludwig DS, Peterson KE, Gortmake SL. "Relation between consumption of sugar-sweetened drinks and childhood obesity: a prospective, observational analysis." *Lancet* 2001;357:505–8.

Nestle, Marion. *Food Politics: How the Industry Influences Nutrition and Health.* Berkeley and Los Angeles, Calif.: University of California Press; London: University of California Press, Ltd., 2002.

Pawlak DB, Kushner JA, Ludwig DS. "Effects of dietary glycaemic index on adiposity, glucose homoeostasis, and plasma lipids in animals." *Lancet* 2004;364:778–85.

Pereira MA, Kartashov AI, Ebbeling CB, et al. "Fast-food habits, weight gain, and insulin resistance (the CARDIA study); 15-year prospective analysis." *Lancet* 2005;365:36–42. (Published erratum appears in *Lancet* 2005 16;365:1030.)

Raben A. Vasilaras TH, Moller AC, Astrup A. "Sucrose compared with artificial sweeteners; different effects on ad libitum food intake and body weight after 10 weeks of supplementation in overweight subjects." *Am J Clin Nutr* 1990;51:963–9.

Rossetti L, Giaccari A, DeFronzo RA. "Glucose toxicity." *Diabetes Care* 1990;13:610–30.

Salmeron J, Manson JE, Stampfer MJ, Colditz GA, Wing AL, Willett WC. "Dietary fiber, glycemic load, and risk of non-insulin-dependent diabetes mellitus in women." *JAMA* 1997;277: 472–7.

Salmeron J, Hu FB, Manson JE, et al. "Dietary fat intake and risk of type 2 diabetes in women." *Am J Clin Nutr* 2001;73:1019–26.

Salmeron J, Ascherio A, Rimm EB, Colditz GA, Spiegelman D, Jenkins DJ. "Dietary fiber, glycemic load, and risk of NIDDM in men." *Diabetes Care* 1997;20:545–50.

Schlosser, Eric. *Fast Food Nation: The Dark Side of the All-American Meal.* New York: HarperCollins, 2002.

Schulze MB, Liu S, Rimm EB, Manson JE, Willett WC, Hu FB. "Glycemic index, glycemic load, and dietary fiber intake and incidence of type 2 diabetes in younger and middle-aged women." *Am J Clin Nutr* 2004;80:348–56.

Schulze MB, Manson JE, Ludwig DS, et al. "Sugar-sweetened beverages, weight gain, and incidence of type 2 diabetes in young and middle-aged women." *JAMA* 2004;292:927–34.

Sears, Barry, with William Lawren. *The Zone: A Dietary Road Map.* New York: HarperCollins, 1995.

Shapiro, Howard M. *Dr. Shapiro's Picture Perfect Weight Loss: The Visual Program for Permanent Weight Loss.* Emmaus, Pa.: Rodale, 2000.

Sinatra, Stephen T. *Optimum Health: A Natural Lifesaving Prescription for Your Body and Mind.* New York: Bantam Books, 1996.

Sinatra, Stephen T., and Jan Sinatra. *Lower Your Blood Pressure in Eight Weeks: A Revolutionary Program for a Longer, Healthier Life.* New York: Ballantine Books, 2003.

Stubbs RJ, Sepp A, Hughes DA, et al. "The effect of graded levels of exercise on energy intake and balance in free-living men, consuming their normal diet." *Eur J Clin Nutr* 2002;56:129–40.

———. "The effect of graded levels of exercise on energy intake and balance in free-living women." *Int J Obes Relat Metab Disord* 2002;26:866–9.

Stubbs RJ, Hughes DA, Johnstone AM, et al. "Rate and extent of compensatory changes in energy intake and expenditure in response to altered exercise and diet composition in humans." *Am J Physiol Regul Integr Comp Physiol* 2004;286:R350–8.

Tordoff MG, Alleva AM. "Effect of drinking soda sweetened with aspartame or high-fructose corn syrup on food intake and body weight." *Am J Clin Nutr* 1990;51:963–9.

van Dam RM, Rimm EB, Willett WC, Stampfer MJ, Hu FB.

"Dietary patterns and risk for type 2 diabetes mellitus in U.S. men." *Ann Intern Med* 2002;136:201–9.

Willett WC, Manson JE, Liu S. "Glycemic index, glycemic load, and risk of type 2 diabetes." *Am J Clin Nutr* 2002;76(suppl): 274S–80S.

Index

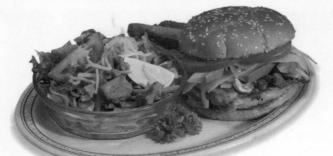

Visit the authors' Web site

Lose Weight, Eat Healthier <u>Without</u> Giving Up Fast Food

Our FREE Website Makes It Easy! Log on today and discover...

- **THE MOST HEALTHFUL MENU ITEMS** for ALL fast food chains and sit-down restaurants in North America

- **20% CASH DISCOUNTS** every time you eat at your favorite fast food and quick dining restaurants

- **MAPPING AND STREET DIRECTIONS** to over 55,000 participating restaurants nationwide

- **ADVANCED ANNOUNCEMENTS** of new menu items

- **FREE WEIGHT-LOSS TIPS** and health advice

- **PERSONAL LOG** of your daily calorie consumptionto keep you on track

- **"QUICK CUISINE"** recipes for nutritious, home-cooked meals

- **OUR "SLIM CHOICE"**™ pick-of-the-day

- **PLUS MANY OTHER FREE FEATURES** that make it easier to lose weight and be healthier

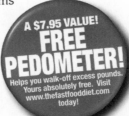

A $7.95 VALUE! **FREE PEDOMETER!** Helps you walk-off excess pounds. Yours absolutely free. Visit www.thefastfooddiet.com today!

www.thefastfooddiet.com

Free pedometers and cash discounts available only while author supply lasts.